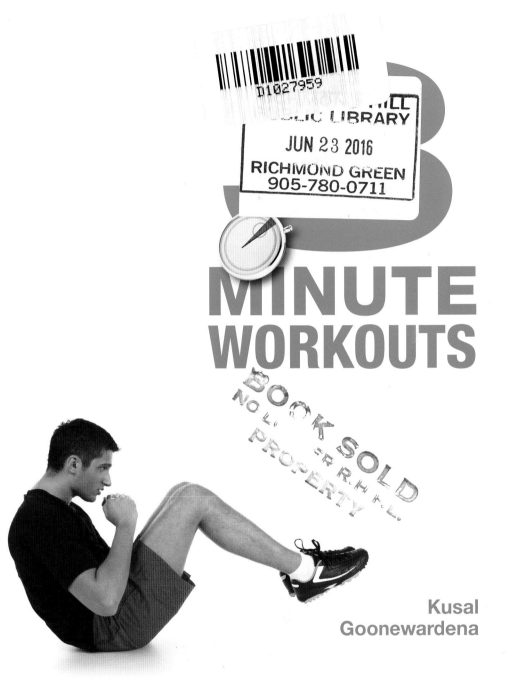

3 MINUTE WORKOUTS

Kusal Goonewardena

WP

WP

Pub...
Wilkinson Publishing Pty L..
ACN 006 042 173
Level 4, 2 Collins Street, Melbourne, Vic 3000
Tel: 03 9654 5446 www.wilkinsonpublishing.com

International distribution by Pineapple Media Ltd
(www.pineapple-media.com) ISSN 2200 -0151

National Library of Australia Cataloguing-in-Publication entry:

Creator: Goonewardena, Kusal, author.

Title: 3 minute workouts / Kusal Goonewardena.

ISBN: 9781925265132 (paperback)

Subjects: Exercise--Popular works.
                  Physical fitness--Popular works.
                  Health--Popular works.

Dewey Number: 615.82

Photos and illustrations by agreement with international agencies,
photographers and illustrators from iStockphoto.
Photos also by agreement with Rodney Stewart.

Design: Jo Hunt
Printed in China

I have so many athletes that travel. They are in and out of hotel rooms, training camps and they live out of their suitcases. I also have so many clients who travel very frequently. Executives, business owners, and CEOs. The commonality between these two diverse groups is that they do not have time to exercise when they want to. They simply do not have time to find the resources (gyms, pools), or they do not have the time to do their exercises.

The 3:21 Routine was created for these people. 3 minutes a day for 21 days straight. For athletes it stopped them from dropping their high standards. For the busy traveller it was perfect to keep in touch with exercises.

Three minutes a day of high intensity exercises for 21 days. No resources required, no sacrifice of time, no finding gyms or pools. The exercises can be done in the comfort of their hotel rooms.

The 3:21 Routine has helped 100s of my clients and athletes. I hope this routine helps you be stronger. I hope it helps you become more active. I hope it opens a door that allows you to exercise more regularly. I hope that the few minutes it takes you to complete the routine provides you with many hours of satisfaction and happiness. I hope the 21 days of exercise will then have your body and mind craving 21 days more. I hope this turns to 3 months of further exercise, activity and sport. I hope this then turns into years of activity that you love. I would be honoured to hear your stories of what you have overcome, what you have endured and how you used exercise to make a difference in your life. My email address: kusal@eliteakademy.com. May this exercise routine be another feather in your cap of exercises.

Wishing you a long, active, happy and satisfied life.

Kusal Goonewardena

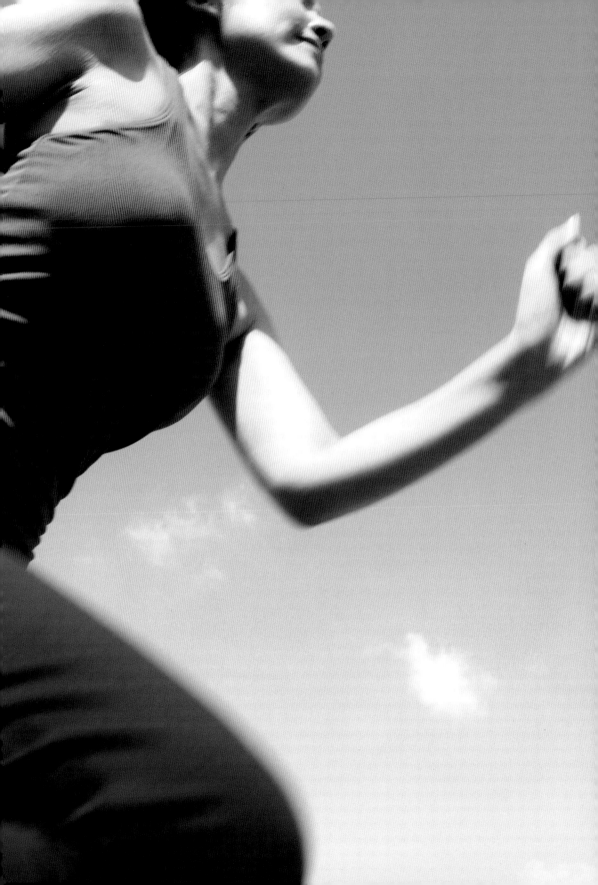

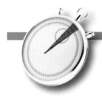

CONTENTS

3 THE AMAZING 3:21 ROUTINE

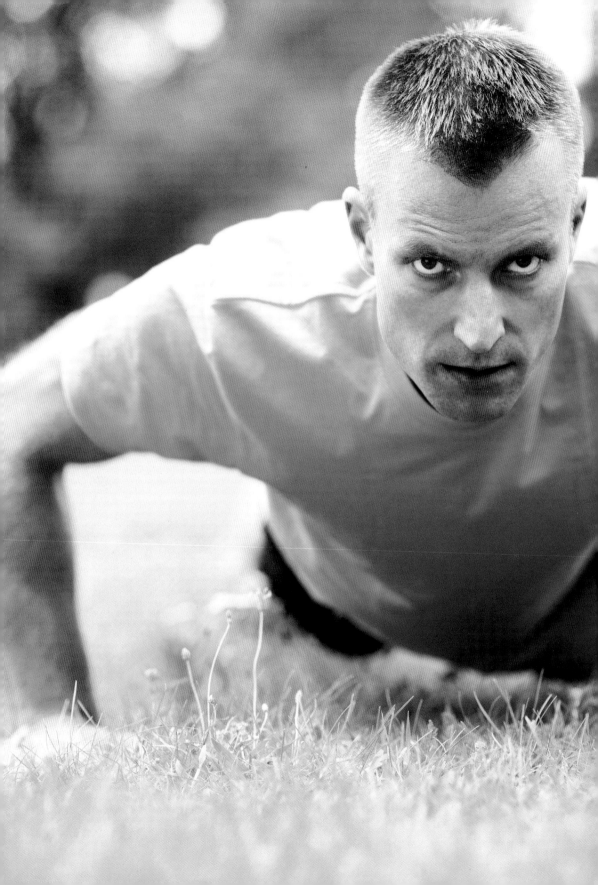

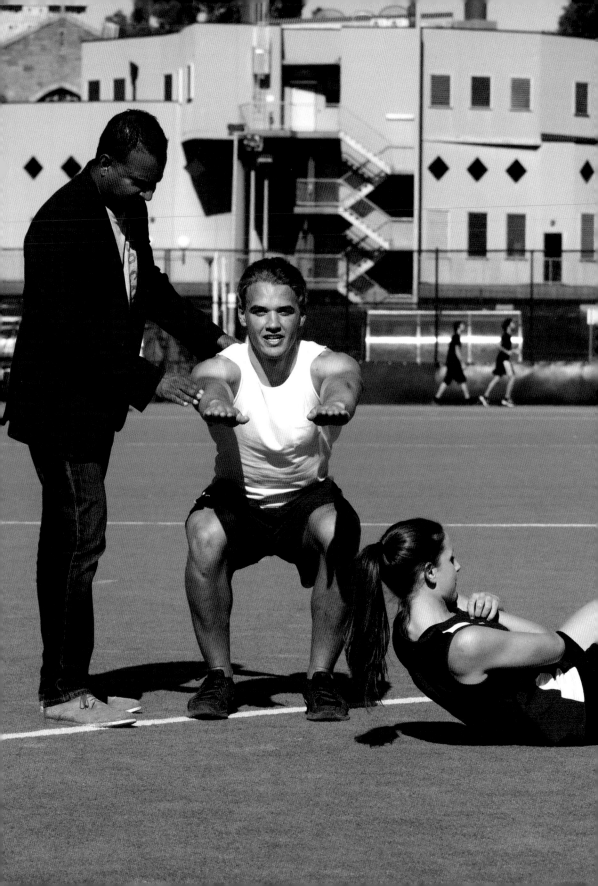

FROM THE AUTHOR'S DESK

Welcome to the world of fitness!

"Give me just 3 minutes a day! I'll prove

I can make you a new person!"

Well said and rightly so! We might hustle around in the clamber to achieve the maximum count of goals and objectives in our lives every day. Stretching our minds and bodies to the fullest, we move on in pursuit of higher gains and richer fames.

The natural mechanism, the wonderful human body, is put to repetitive tests and trials in this entire flurry. With all its amazing systems and organs, the body dutifully continues to churn out results, one after the other. In this process, the internal systems undergo a vast series of wear and tear, along with often irreparable damages to some of its most crucial wings.

Here, what we need to ponder is what is it that actually fuels the body's wear and tear, it's constant operation and the works? Is it food, sleep or exercise?

Well, let's find out!

The human body is comprised of a series of body systems, ranging right from the all-important cardiovascular and nervous systems to the more silent ones like the circulatory system. Now, all of them work in tandem and the functioning of one affects the other. What, we, as mortal laypeople often don't realize is that beyond the basics of food and sleep, there is another important element that keeps it all going. This mystical element is nothing else but the all-powerful streak of energy which flows all over our body that rejuvenates the whole mechanism and actually gives 'life' to life.

To achieve the purpose of our life and to scale the desired heights, it is important that we keep this wave of energy in its peak form, fueling it with whatever it takes to keep the flow of energy going.

You can enjoy the exercise routines in this book and if you wish for a challenge set out by the author go here.

The 3 Minute Workout Challenge
www.eliteakademy.com/3-minute-challenge

This will help you go to the next level!

The 3:21 program, the focus and epicenter of this book does just that! It gives you a practical and abridged, but powerful, capsule to keep this flow of energy intact.

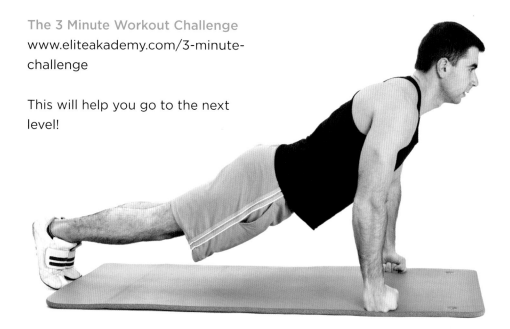

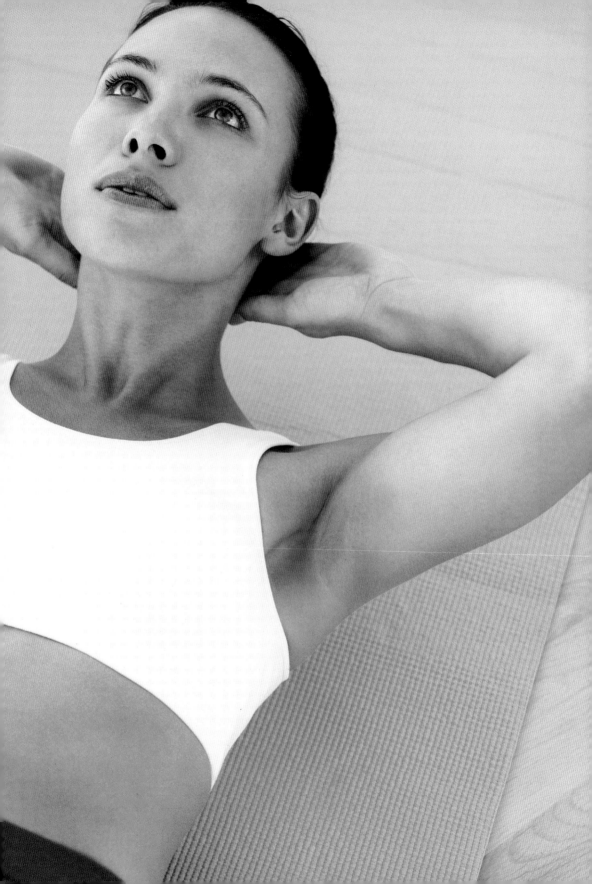

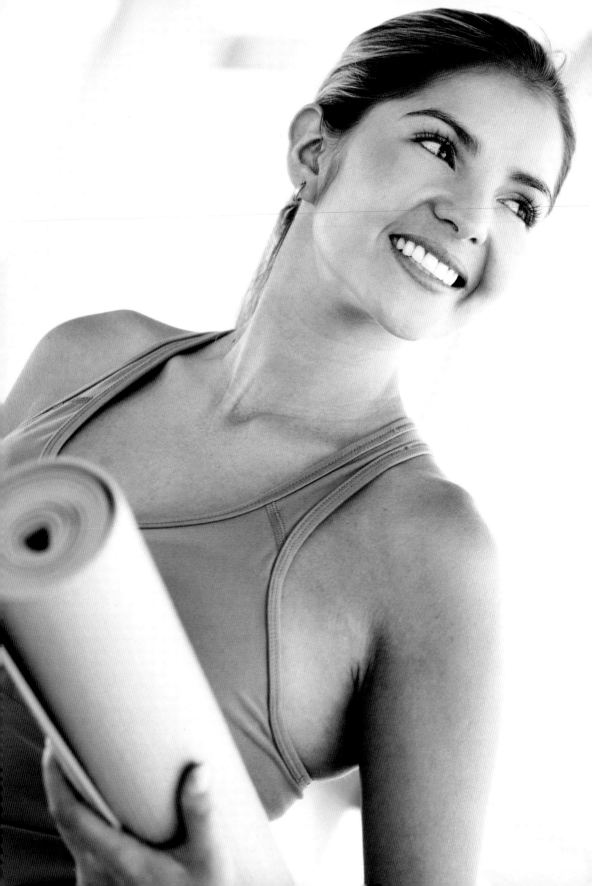

1

THE WORLD OF WORKOUTS

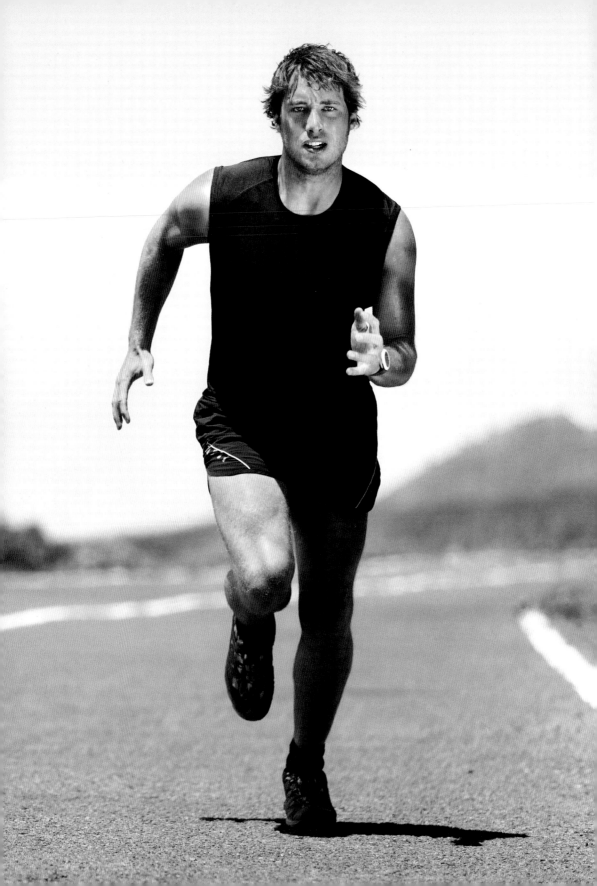

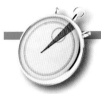

WHY EXERCISE?

Take care of your body. It's the only place you have to live!

JIM ROHN

The human body is indeed an amazing mechanism. Like a sophisticated automobile, it has zillions of components, processes and parts working in tandem to make us breathe, work and live.

Unfortunately, the similarity ends here!

Let's ponder over a question here, before we move on! What do you do when your favorite car or bike keeps breaking down? Obviously, you take it to the suitable workshop and get the erratic parts mended. After your car has had too many troubles, you finally bid it farewell and walk to the showroom for a shining new vehicle. Your issues stand solved.

Sadly enough, the same is not the case with our bodies. No doubt science and technology has given us an amazing array of health benefits and options and right from a knee to kidneys and even the heart, everything can be transplanted.

However, Mother Nature still retains its right to take the final call here. There comes a point when all the medical advances fail to help you, if you've spoiled your body's original balance. Not everything in the world is replaceable. Once the body sets on the path of deterioration, the drive is often uphill, in spite of the best of resources and care being at your disposal.

Just remember, no amount of medical care will help you if you have not adhered to the basic dictums of good health, which are:

✓ **Regular exercise**

✓ **Right diet**

✓ **Healthy lifestyle**

Frustrating as it might sound, even if one of the above is left out, our body spirals out of its natural balance. It is this imbalance that leads to disease, sickness and ill-health.

Isn't it time you took charge of your body, mind and health?

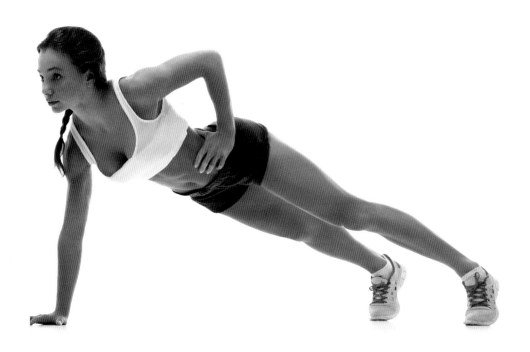

THE WORLD'S FITNESS CRISIS

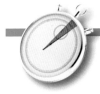

Lifestyles have changed and so has the quality of food available to us. The effort that traditionally used to go into preparing daily meals has reduced to a great extent. Meanwhile, our sedentary habits have taken over. From climbing stairs, we've moved on to elevators and from walking even shorter distances, we don't mind using our luxury cars!

Strange, isn't it? Modern developments and technological advancement made by man have ended up posing a serious threat to his health in return!

Hence, here comes the Workout Revolution! With all our fancy resources, we've now moved on to building great resources for maintaining our fitness levels.

Research shows at least a modest 132 million of the world's population are associated with a health club, fitness centre or a gym.

Also, just imagine the 8.1 percent rate of growth in the revenue from fitness sector, happening in the US every year!

Age, gender, occupation being no bar, individuals from all cross-sections of society are now taking to serious fitness planning for the sake of their health.

Here, let's take a look at the main forms of exercise and workouts that rule the roost, being adopted by the majority of people today. Each of these exercises has its own set of workouts, with each having their own advantages and drawbacks.

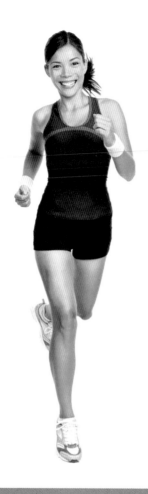

ANAEROBIC EXERCISES

✓ Intensity: Moderate to high

✓ Key benefit: Encourages power, muscle build-up and maximum oxygen consumption

✓ Prominent examples: Strength exercises, with/ without equipment

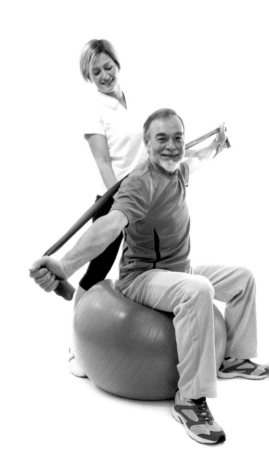

AEROBIC EXERCISES

✓ Intensity: Moderate

✓ Key benefit: Promotes good cardiovascular health

✓ Prominent examples: Walking, cycling, running, hiking, jogging

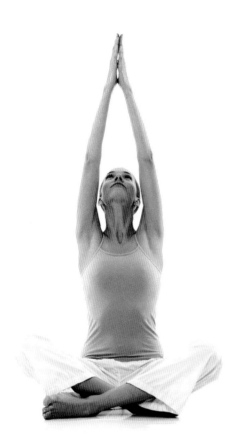

THE MINIMUM REQUIREMENT

So, what is the minimum requirement for the amount of exercise you should be doing to stay fit and healthy?

Well, as per experts, a normal, healthy person should take up at least 2.5 hours of physical activity of moderate intensity (such as walking) per week. Alternatively, one can also take up 1.5 hours of vigorous exercise (such as swimming or jogging), supplemented by at least 2 sessions of muscle-strengthening exercises every week. It is the latter option which is gaining immense popularity in today's generation, the reasons and explanation or which you will read in the coming sections.

FLEXIBILITY EXERCISES

✓ Intensity: Moderate

✓ Key benefit: Improves range of motion of muscles, joints and ligaments

✓ Prominent examples: Stretches and yoga We shall read more about these exercises in the coming chapters.

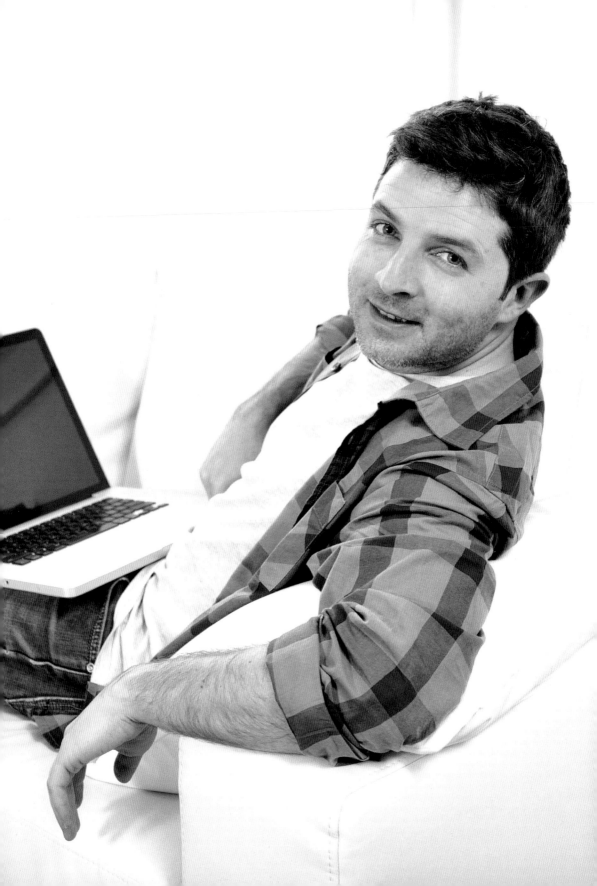

THE 5 ROADBLOCKS

Getting comfortable by being uncomfortable..... that's exercise!

With such clarity on the need of exercise and workouts, the glaring lack of a proper fitness routine in an average individual's life is quite surprising. Finances notwithstanding, even people with the best of resources and time are failing to hit the gym or go for that often postponed walk, in spite of the medics shouting warning signs. Just consider the damage you'll be doing to your body!

Before we go any further, let's just look in to the reasons and roadblocks that prevent most of the population from taking up exercise regularly.

1 Lack of motivation

Sadly enough, even after being fully aware of the consequences, a majority of the people fall victim to physical inactivity. It is a little surprise then that reports state physical inactivity to be the fourth leading risk factor contributing to global mortality and leading to almost 3.2 million deaths annually, across the world. The very motivation to leave our comfort zone and push our body to exert is missing and is often hard to get. Unfortunately, the more we get into our comfort zones, the tougher it is to get out and start exercising.

2 Lack of time

The flurry to achieve more leaves little time for exercise and workout. It is often seen that most of the people recognize the need to remain fit long after the damage has already been done. Given that most of the steady-state workouts usually take a lot of time, this indeed is one of the major reasons. It is for this paucity of time that the short, high intensity workouts have come to rule the world of fitness today. We'll read more on it in the coming chapters.

3 Lack of knowledge and resources

It is a fact that even 15 minutes a day can do wonders for your fitness levels if the right workouts are done for your body. Often, we don't know what kind of exercises need to be done and end up spending futile minutes and hours of exertion and sweat. It is important to exercise under the guidance or supervision of an appropriate guide or instructor to achieve best results.

4 Imbalanced results

It often happens that an improper technique combined with wrong exercises mostly have the opposite effect than desired. When we get into such a situation, it is very natural to get deterred from exercising in the future as well. The most common sentiment in this situation is that probably exercising is not right for you and so on.

5 Lack of funds

Membership of health clubs and gymnasiums often come at exorbitant prices. Even personal trainers prove to be quite expensive most of the times. It is for these reasons that most of the individuals often shy away from exercising. In times when a majority of the families face a financial crunch, spending on fitness and exercises might come across as futile to most of us.

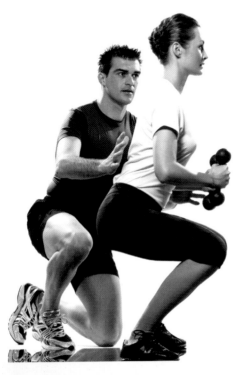

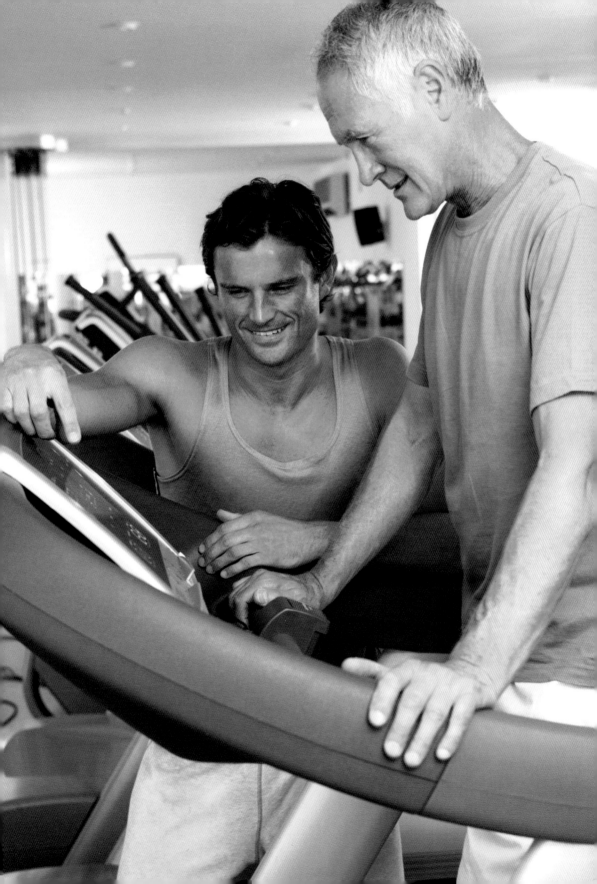

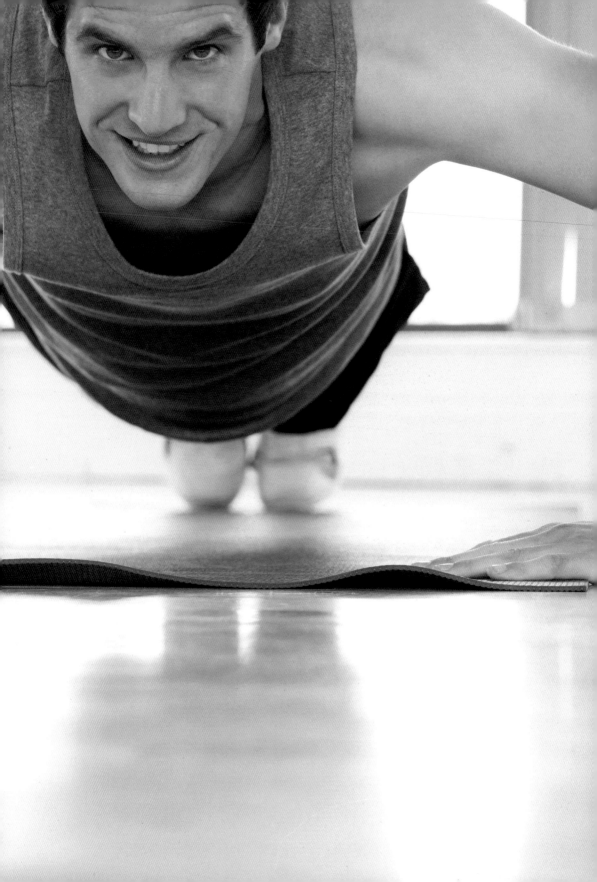

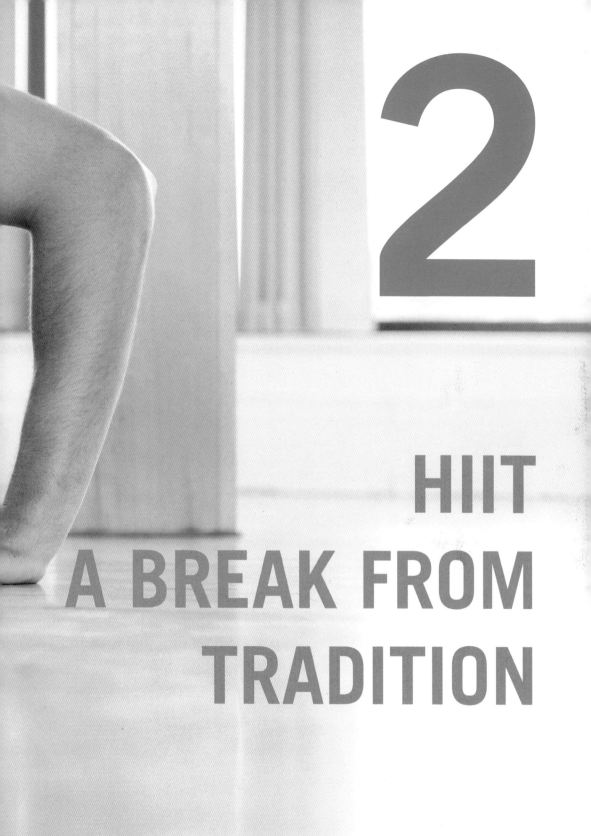

2

HIIT
A BREAK FROM TRADITION

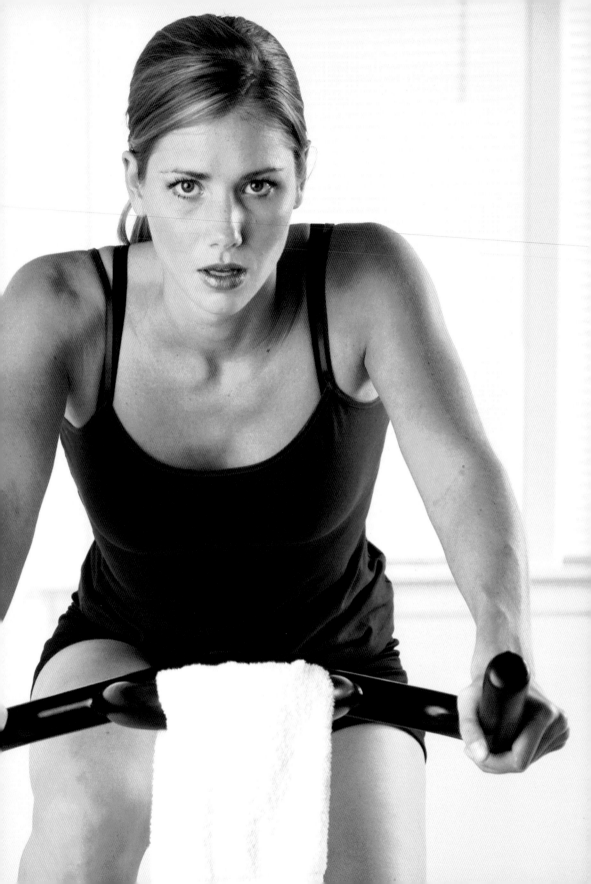

ALL ABOUT HIIT

"But, where is the time?"

This oft-heard and quoted question finally takes a beat with the new trend of short, power-packed, high intensity workouts. Designed to fit in snuggly with the busy routines of the modern day life, these workouts have almost changed the way we've seen fitness across the years.

A conventional fitness program would usually span across at least a 45-minute session each, for minimum of 5 days a week. It would comprise of a wide range of activities to make an ideal fitness plan in those days. As it is evident, quite a few people have eventually started finding this mode of exercise to be very tedious and time-consuming. Fitness scientists and experts around the world have started research on abridging the standard workout, keeping the goodness intact.

It was then that the world started taking notice of the new power-packed High Intensity Interval Training (HIIT), the professionally designed and shortened fitness capsules. With the packages promising to offer the same or even better impact in as much as a one-third of the usual time, the HIIT surely made its inroads into the fitness industry in a remarkable span of time. In the following sections, you will read all about HIIT, right from the basics, the concept, its benefits, the schedules and most importantly, just how the HIIT is more beneficial in the modern times.

THE BASICS

The High Intensity Interval Training (HIIT) is a typical, conceptual shift from the original form of aerobics, anaerobic and other workouts. It shifts the focus of fitness away from duration and brings the intensity and method of exercise into the spotlight. Experts define HIIT as an innovative cardio training schedule, in which two types of modules or sessions are done in an alternate manner, which include:

✓ **Short duration, very high intensity exercise modules**

✓ **Short intervals of moderate activity or rest**

In spite of its vast array of benefits, experts do point out that the high intensity exercise might not suit everyone. Just make sure that you have right level of fitness and health to begin the strong regimen. For instance, HIIT is not recommended for you if you have a heart condition or have suffered from joint or musculoskeletal injuries in the recent past.

HIIT is a professionally designed system of cardio respiratory training which has short, high intensity bouts of exercise, intermingled with brief periods of low level of activity with lesser exertion or even rest.

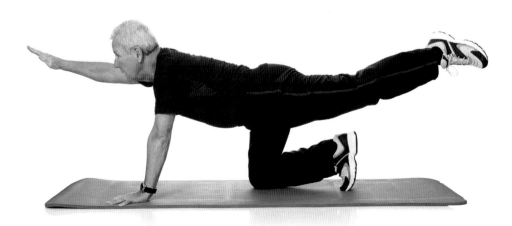

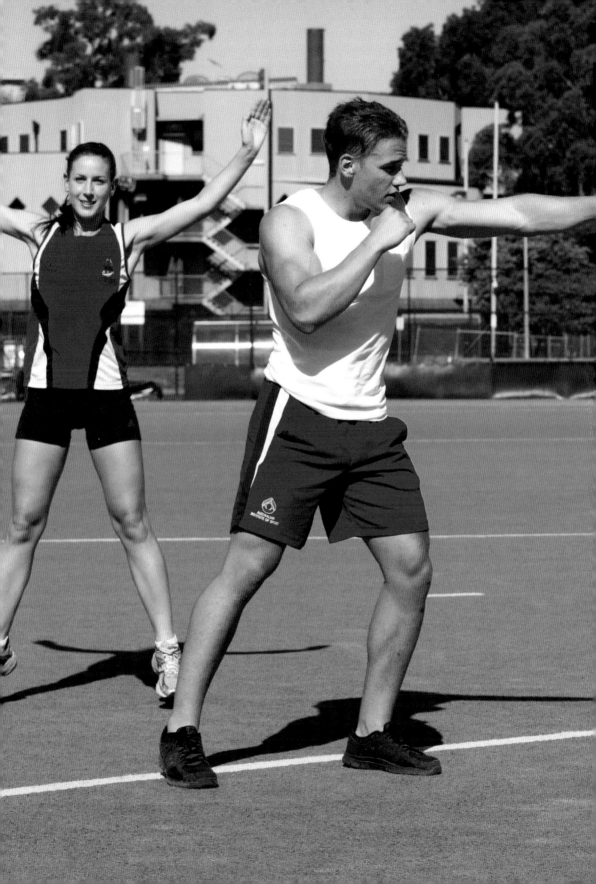

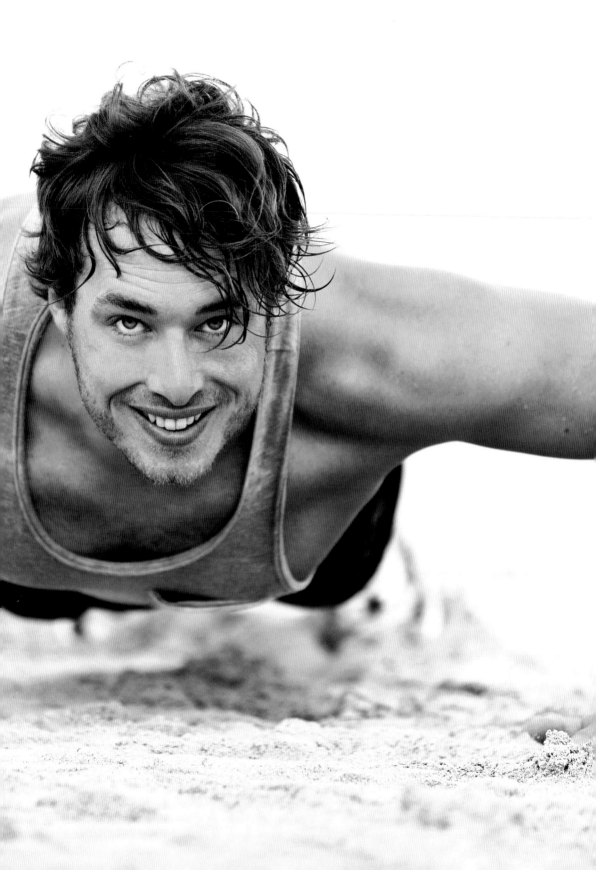

HIGH INTENSITY EXERCISE – THE PARAMETERS

The intensity of exercise defines the very basis of a High Intensity Interval Training Schedule.

Let's understand a bit more about what actually defines high intensity before we move ahead. According to the American Council of Exercise (ACE), there are two broad parameters that define the intensity of your exercise, including:

✓ **Level of effort**

✓ **Level of your Maximum Heart Rate (MHR)**

Each of them is explained below in detail.

Level of effort

For the purpose of understanding, just rate the amount of effort that goes into physical exercise from 1 to 10, with 1 being the point of least effort. High intensity exercise actually takes place when you exert to anything more than the level of 7.

Maximum heart rate (MHR)

Similarly, we can also understand this concept using the scale of maximum heart rate (MHR). Heart rate is the typical speed of your heartbeat or the number of heartbeats per a specific unit of time. The unit of measurement used for Heart Rate is beats per minute (bpm). This heart rate varies in accordance with the body's physical needs, primarily including the need to absorb oxygen and expel carbon dioxide. Exercise is one of the most important factors that can influence your heart rate.

Meanwhile, the MHR is the highest level of heart rate an individual can achieve without causing serious problems.

You can know that you are doing high intensity exercise when your MHR goes beyond 80%. Refer to the diagram below to understand the parameters better.

THE BREATH TEST

This is a simpler method of measuring your level of intensity. Try to talk and make small conversation while exercising. If you are being able to talk comfortably and are fairly audible, your level of exercise would be termed as moderate. However, you are doing intense exercise if you barely manage to form a sentence and feel breathless as you attempt to talk.

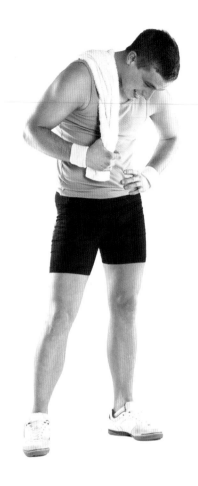

HIIT – THE PARAMETERS

Scale of Effort

							HIIT		
1	2	3	3	5	6	7	8	9	10

Max Heart Rate (MHR)   50%   80%   HIIT

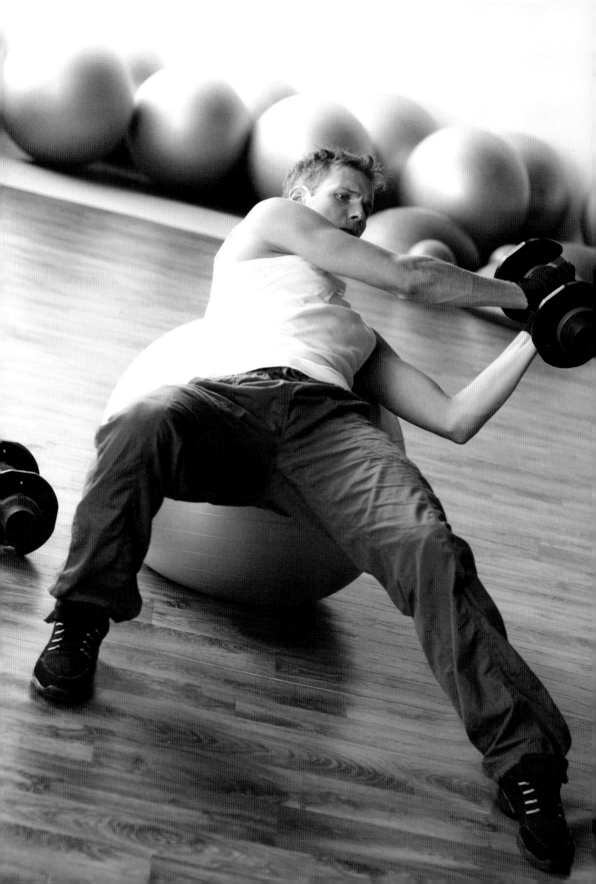

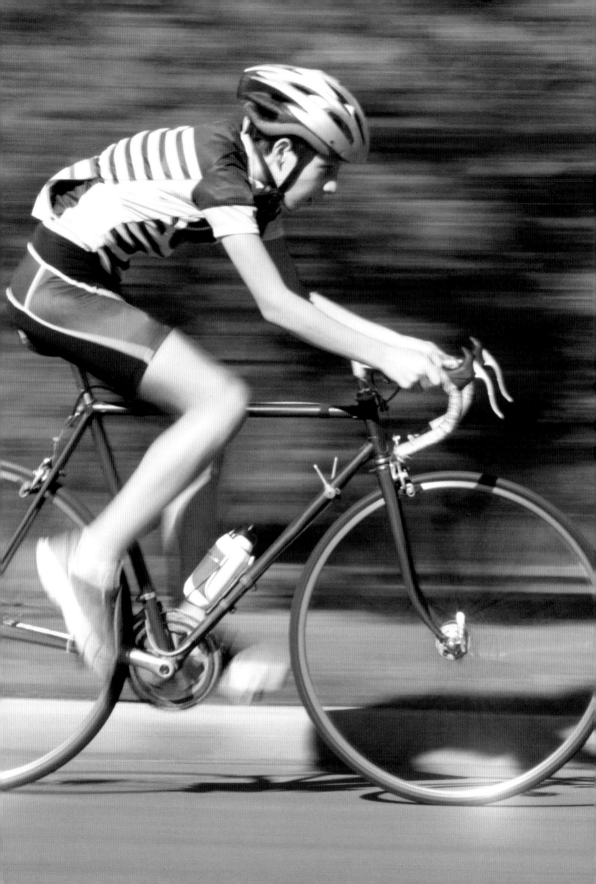

AEROBICS VS. ANAEROBICS

Before we study the underlying logic of HIIT in detail, let's first understand what exactly do aerobics and anaerobic exercises mean.

Aerobic exercises – the endurance training regimen

The term aerobic literally means 'relating to, involving or requiring free oxygen'. A typical aerobic exercise promotes the circulation of oxygen through the blood and enhances the rate of breathing. When we indulge in aerobics, our body procures the oxygen from the air and transfers it from the lungs to the blood and muscles through the circulatory system. Put simply, aerobic exercise, also known as cardiovascular exercise is just a muscle movement that will use oxygen to burn carbohydrates and fats to produce energy. A typical aerobic exercise plan is aimed at increasing your level of endurance.

An individual's aerobic fitness would be defined as the ability to take oxygen from the atmosphere and use it to produce energy for your muscle cells. A typical measure of your aerobic fitness would be Maximal Aerobic Power or Maximal Oxygen Uptake, also known as VO2Max. Some of the factors that might influence your aerobic fitness include:

✓ **Lung efficiency**

✓ **Cardiac Function**

✓ **Gender**

✓ **Age**

✓ **Training schedule and status**

✓ **Genetic makeup**

Some of the most common forms of aerobic exercises include:

✓ **Running**

✓ **Jogging**

✓ **Swimming**

✓ **Cycling**

Just as a reference, HIIT basically involves pushing you way beyond your upper aerobic exercise zone.

Anaerobic exercises – the strength training regimen

The term anaerobic literally means 'without air'.

Anaerobic exercise is typically defined as a muscle movement that does not require oxygen and will burn the carbohydrates to produce energy.

Put in other words, anaerobic exercises are short duration, high intensity exercises where your body's demand for oxygen will be more than its supply, thereby creating a major oxygen deficit. The aim of a typical anaerobic exercise would be build muscle and increase physical strength.

Some of the most typical forms of anaerobic exercise include:

✓ **Weightlifting**

✓ **Push-ups**

✓ **Sit-ups**

✓ **Sprinting**

✓ **Jumping**

The scientific measure of anaerobic fitness is the anaerobic threshold (AT), which is the exercise intensity at which lactate or lactic acid starts to accumulate in the blood stream. In a normal exercise module that happens below the AT threshold, lactate is produced by the muscles effectively, before allowing to build it up.

It is by the effective combination of the strengths of both, the aerobics and anaerobic exercises, that a typical, result-oriented HIIT module is designed.

In the next section, we will explain the underlying logic of the HIIT module in detail.

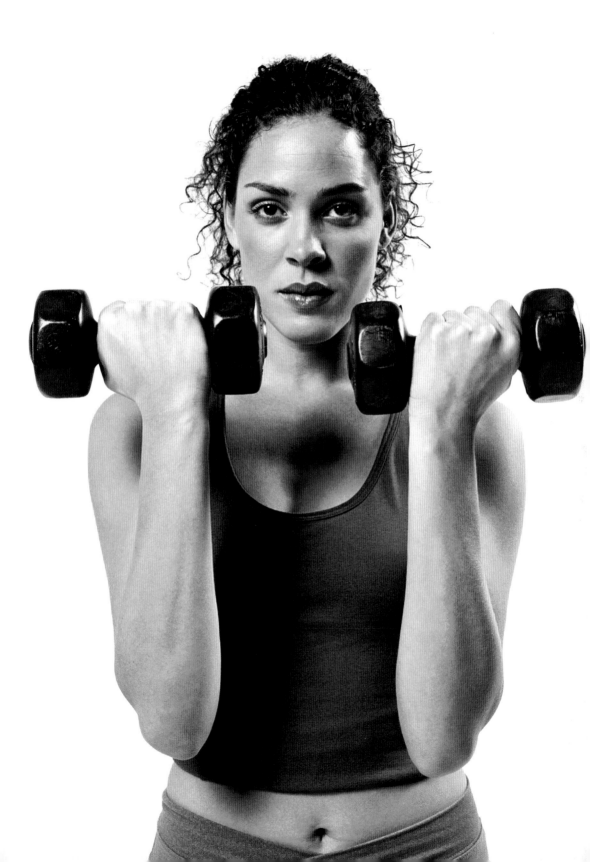

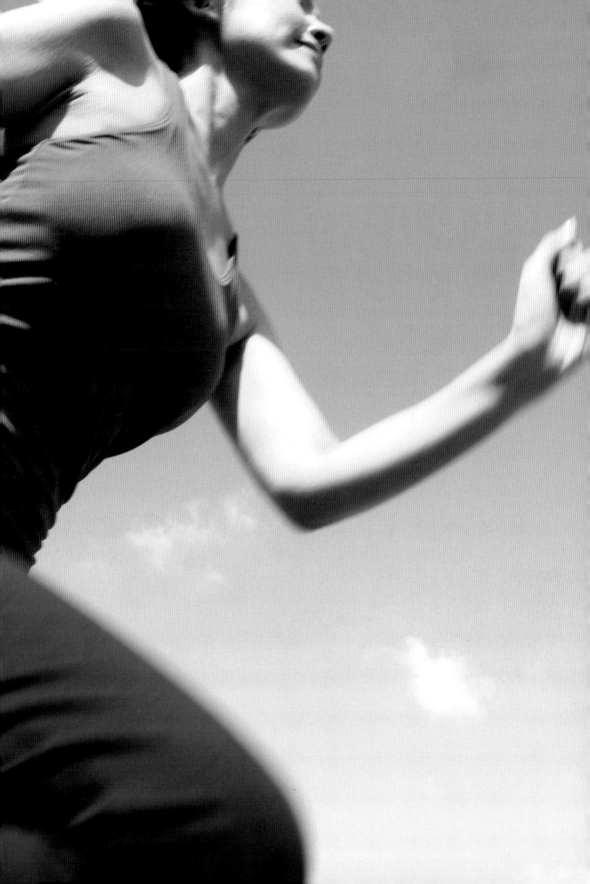

HIIT -
THE LOGIC

To understand how HIIT works, let's look at some of the most important aspects of the key underlying logic of the exercise routine.

Heart rate

When we exercise, we usually choose to work out to the level in which our heart rate stays within our aerobic zone. In laymen terms, this implies that we workout to the limit our body physically allows us to. However, with HIIT, we push our body way beyond our upper aerobic zone. This brings us to the first key logic of HIIT. Though it might appear so, HIIT not only causes a higher heart rate, but also involves maximum effort, beyond our conventional limits.

Types of muscles used

The second logic of HIIT lies within the type of muscle fibers used. Due to it's format, HIIT uses large and strong muscle fibers that would otherwise lie dormant during the conventional steady-state exercises.

Oxygen consumption and calories burnt

The third and most important logic that explains the momentous success of HIIT lies in the concept of oxygen consumption by our body. During a steady-state exercise, our body only requires a limited amount of oxygen since we are exercising within our aerobic zone. However, during a HIIT schedule, the demand of oxygen goes way beyond its supply, thereby creating an oxygen deficit.

Hence, our body continues to burn calories even in the rest periods after the exercise. While such a period of burning calories can last for hours after a HIIT session, a similar effect lasts for only a few minutes after a standard steady-state exercise routine.

The Flow of Energy

By now, we know how the HIIT effectively combines the regimens of aerobics and anaerobic workout. The flow of energy in both these workouts can also help us understand the underlying logic of HIIT better.

As we indulge in an aerobic workout, our body produces oxygen from the atmosphere, which then gets circulated into our blood and energy system from the lungs. Meanwhile, your body also learns to create and utilize the energy that comes from its anaerobic energy system.

THE COMPONENTS

A typical HIIT schedule will have almost equal sets of high intensity and low-effort exercise modules. Ideally, a HIIT schedule will have 30-second to 3-minute intervals of high intensity cardiovascular exercise, alternating with varying periods of low intensity or rest.

Some of the most typical components of a HIIT schedule include:

✓ **Treadmills**

✓ **Elliptical runners**

✓ **Stair climbers**

✓ **Stationery bikes**

✓ **Sprints**

Interestingly, HIIT experts point out that apart from the structured activities, you can perform any of your daily physical activities in the manner of HIIT. For instance, even playing throw and chase ball with your dog can be a form of HIIT, if done actively adding variety to your routine.

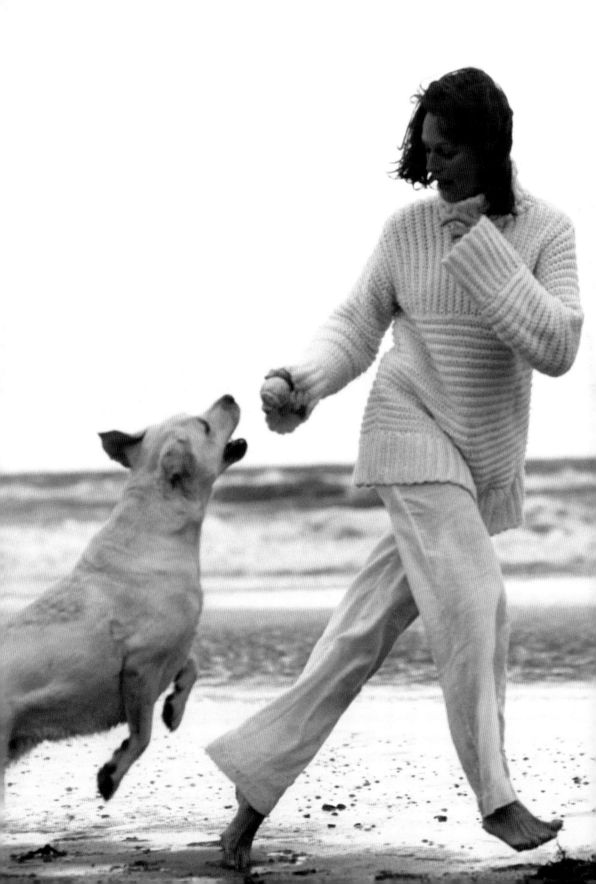

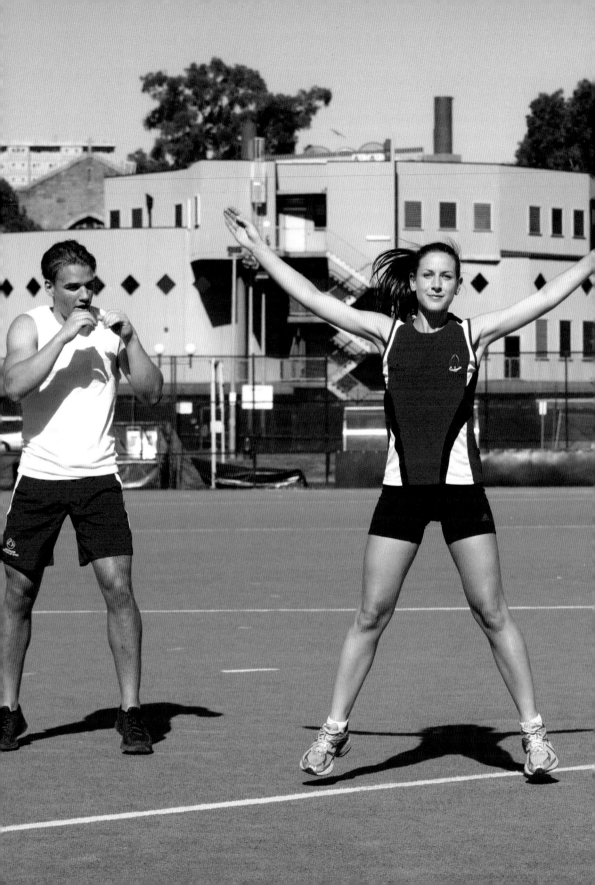

THE 15 TOP BENEFITS

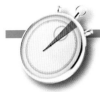

The world has been taken by storm by the onslaught of the miracle capsule of HIIT, owing to its staggering range of benefits. Such a high intensity workout when combined with brief intervals of low effort exercise help in increasing metabolic functioning. The methodology also helps in promoting fat loss.

The latest research also shows that that high-intensity, interval training is one of the best ways to get into shape and lose fat. In fact, a relevant research published in the *Journal of Obesity* actually showed that 12 weeks of HIIT can lead to substantive reductions in trunk, abdominal and visceral fat, apart from increasing your fat-free mass and aerobic ability.

Just remember!

The HIIT routine should never be mistaken as the easier way out! It is just less time consuming, with quicker results...but not as easy to do....

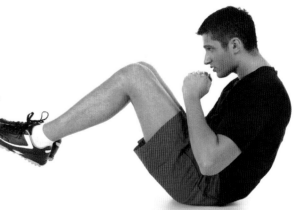

Here, we've discussed and listed some of the most important benefits and advantages of doing a High Intensity Interval Training program.

1 Time is the biggest factor. A 30-minute HIIT session is likely to have a similar impact as a 90-minute low-intensity session. Similarly, 15 minutes of interval training done thrice a week will have more visible results than jogging on the treadmill for an hour every day. Hence, the time factor is one of the most important benefits.

2 Minimal equipment and structured space is required for doing HIIT.

3 We've seen how HIIT involves the regimen of anaerobic exercises as well. It can effectively train the body to produce and use the energy from the anaerobic energy system.

4 The amount of oxygen consumed in HIIT is much higher than standard, steady-state exercises. This higher rate in turn increases your metabolism rate from 90 minutes to 2.4 hours per each session of HIIT. Eventually, the higher metabolism helps your body to burn the fat and calories much faster.

5 The short intervals of moderate activity or rest help in removing the metabolic waste from the muscles.

6 As per the relevant research, HIIT training gives a considerable boost to the Human Growth Hormone (HGH), also known as the fitness hormone, almost by a whopping 450 percent in the first 24 hours. The HGH actually offers you the twin benefit of lowering the aging process and increasing the rate at which calories are burnt.

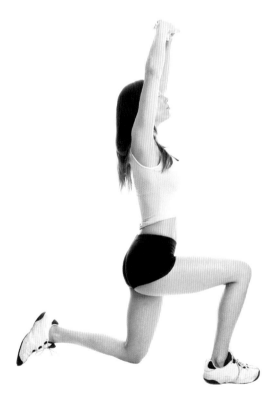

7 HIIT also has potential benefits for healthy but physically inactive people. Short but intense bouts of exercise in such people actually led to a measurable change in their DNA, reflecting to the power the workout has.

8 It increases the amount of calories burnt during and after the exercise, since your body keeps burning calories even after the workout is over.

9 HIIT increases the time span your body requires to recover from each session. Due to this, your body keeps burning more calories even after the workout is over.

10 HIIT is suspected to be helpful in improving insulin sensitivity in the muscles.

11 There can be a drastic increase in the stamina levels. A random study amongst cyclists revealed that those who participated in a HIIT program for 8 weeks could easily spend double the time on their bikes at the same pace.

12 The alternating format of HIIT helps you to maximize the volume of air that is inhaled during a workout.

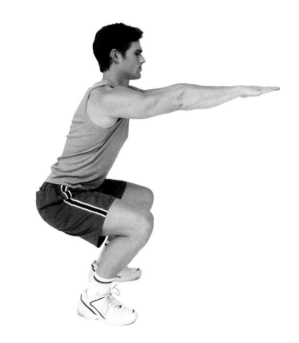

13 HIIT is also known to reducing aortic stiffness that affects how quickly blood travels through the arteries.

14 Helps reduce chances of heart disease, hypertension and diabetes.

15 Most of the modules in HIIT are functional in nature. This means that by performing these exercises on a regular basis, you are able to perform your routine activities with a greater ease. For instance, performing squat jumps makes squatting easier and more comfortable and even improves the functioning of your excretory system.

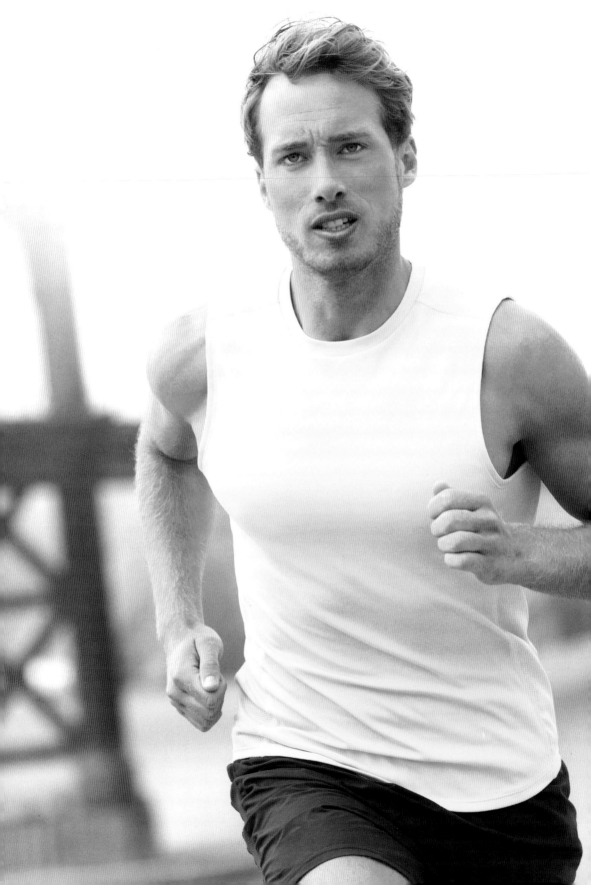

THE 5 NEW-WORLD PROBLEMS SOLVED

By now, we've read and studied all about HIIT, its underlying logic and key benefits. Having understood the theoretical part, let's move on to see how exactly HIIT promises to solve the 5 most critical fitness issues faced by the modern world. In this section, we will talk about the 5 most serious problems and deterrents that discourage people from exercising and how HIIT addresses these concerns effectively.

1 It handles your time crunch

Repetitive research churns out impressive figures on how HIIT manages to give you the same results as a steady-state exercise would, in less than half the time. Shorter bouts of higher intensity in interval training compete very well with longer, tedious sessions of slow and steady exercise in all aspects such as weight loss, muscle toning, and fat reduction and so on.

2 It keeps you motivated with variety and no pre-requisites

Today's world likes fast-paced and innovative activities. Though patience is still very much a virtue, it is very easy to lose interest long-winded, similar exercise routines to be done every day. HIIT offers an almost unlimited array of workouts you can do, even turning your everyday jobs into periods of high intensity exercise. A few common examples include a fast jog when taking your dog for a walk, short sprints on a holiday and so on.

Moreover, for a steady-state exercise, we usually get discouraged if we would have to go searching for formal equipment or a structured space. With almost no such pre-requisite for HIIT, there is nothing much dampening your spirit to do your workout!

3 It burns more calories

Earlier in this book, we've explained how your body burns more calories during a HIIT workout. However, what is more important is that your body continues to burn calories even in the hours after the workout in order to meet the heightened demand for oxygen. This alters your metabolic rate in a beneficial way, while keeping the calorie count well in control. The result here is higher amounts of calories burnt in a lesser amount of time, with the effect lingering on after your workout is over.

4 It doesn't cause muscle loss

HIIT promotes good muscle health which is very important in today's sedentary lifestyles. First of all, it uses a lot of muscle fibers which would otherwise lie dormant during a conventional workout. Besides, a typical HIIT routine will help you lose weight without causing excessive muscle loss, which will prevent further complications like sagging of the skin and so on.

The table at the end of this section gives a quick comparative summary of the traditional steady state exercises and HIIT.

5 It gives you the correct way to exercise

Even proper exercise, with ample time and resources fails to give you the desired results. It often happens that we exercise without any pre-designed program and end up frustrated and confused. HIIT give you the right direction, telling you how to exercise, how much time to devote and most important of all, which exercises suit your body type the most.

HIIT Vs. Steady-State Exercises

TRADITIONAL STEADY-STATE EXERCISES	HIIT
Time-consuming and tedious	Takes less than half the time, producing similar results
Can turn monotonous and hence, de-motivating	Offers a lot of variety and hence keeps the motivation alive
Burns only fats within the body	Also burns the carbohydrates stored in the body
Burns calories only during the workout	Burns calories even after the workout is over
Burns limited calories during the workout	Burns higher amount of calories during the workout
Might cause muscle loss along with weight/fat loss	Avoids muscle loss associated with weight loss
Equipment is usually required	No equipment necessary
Structured space is required	Can be done anywhere, in as much time as you have

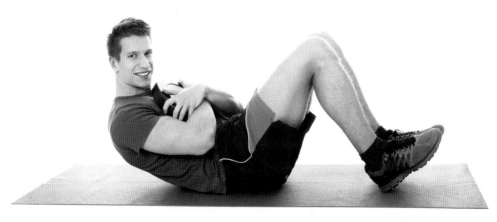

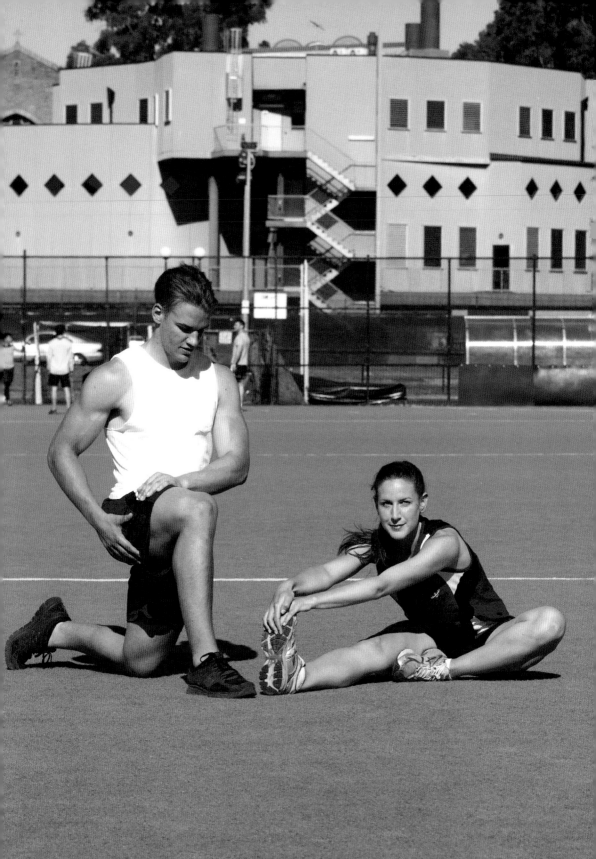

HIIT – THE FAQS

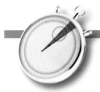

With so many amazing benefits around it, a module such as the HIIT is bound to be laden with doubts. In this section, we answer some of the most often asked questions related to the HIIT programs.

The basic of value of a HIIT program lies in its suitability to a wide range of people.

1 Who can do it?

The basic of value of a HIIT program lies in its suitability to a wide range of people. There are a few prominent factors that determine whether a particular individual is eligible for adopting a HIIT plan. The most important factor here is the state of fitness. It is important for an individual to have at least a moderate fitness level. The concerned person should be performing at least some amount of exercise on a routine basis. This is important because to do a HIIT regimen, the basic flexibility in the muscles and ligaments should be there. Certain injuries or problems might occur if an absolute novice to exercise starts on a HIIT program straightaway.

2 When will I see the results?

Well, it again depends on your current level of fitness. If you are already fit and toned enough, the HIIT program will begin to show instantaneous results. However, if your body is not in a very fit condition, it might take time for the results to show. Your body will first try to adapt to the regime, the muscles will get into shape and then the actual results will begin to show.

3 How is it possible?

The human body follows a certain pattern in which it burns calories and facilitates weight loss. In an HIIT program, third pattern undergoes a major change as the calories are now burnt at a faster rate. What's more, your body also continues to burn calories much after the workout is over. All of this has a compound effect on your body, which in turn effects how fast you lose weight and get into shape, as promised by a HIIT program.

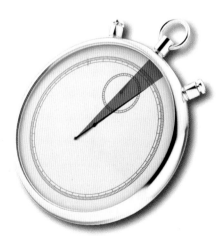

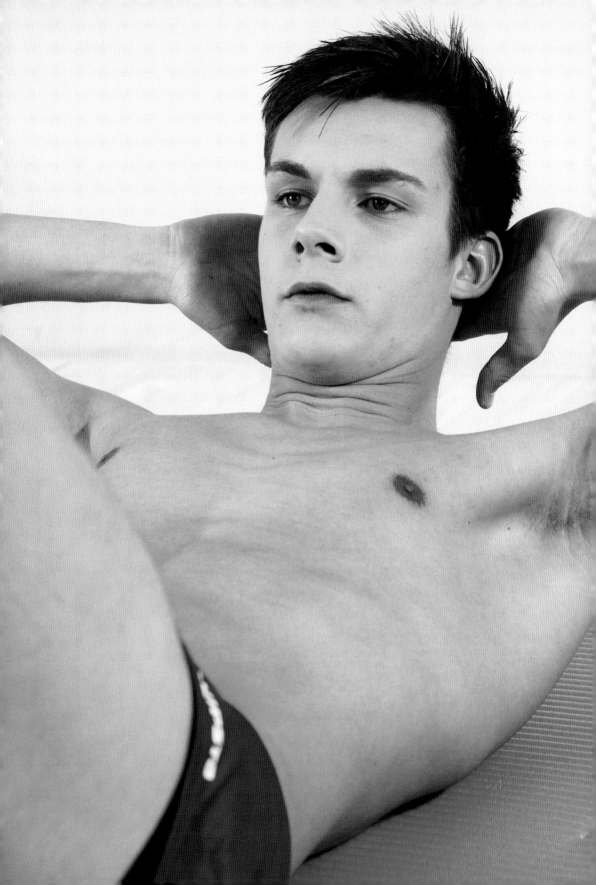

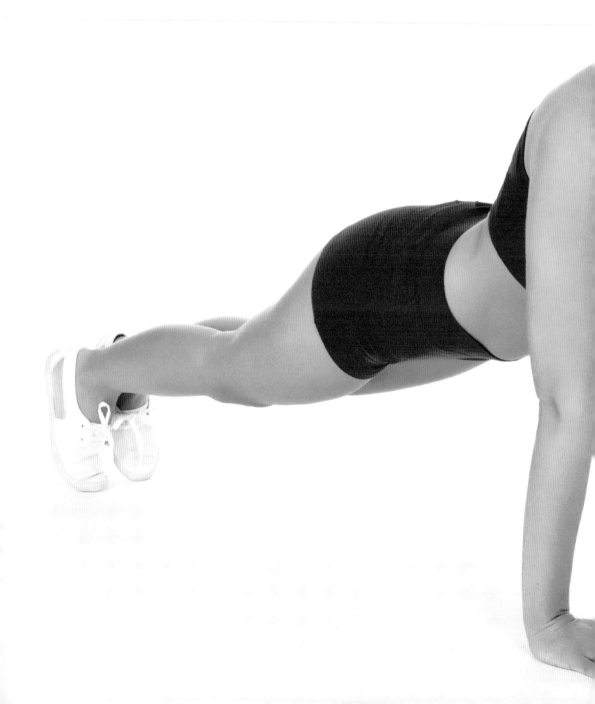

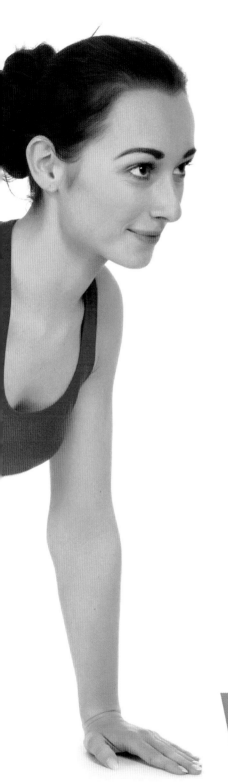

3

THE AMAZING 3:21 WORKOUT

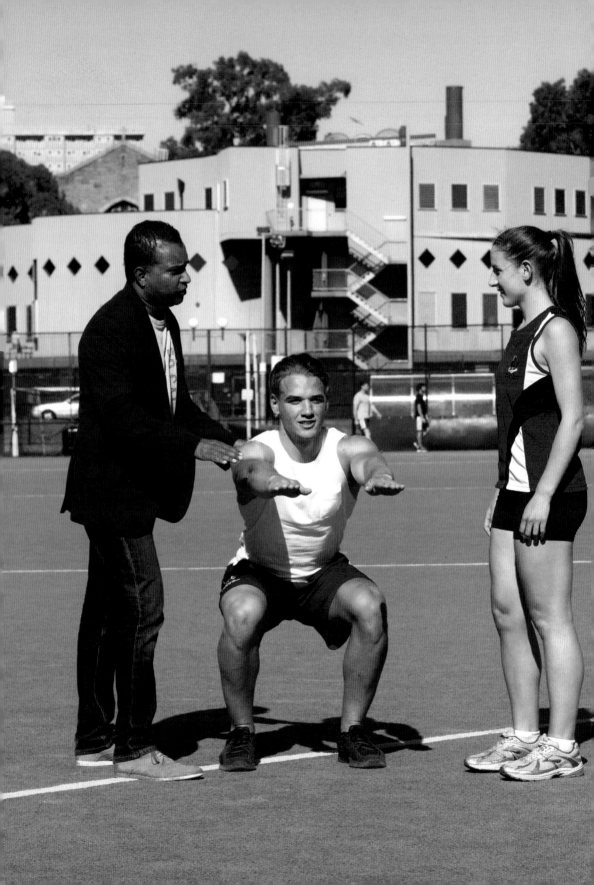

FOUNDER - THE ELITE SPORTS PHYSIOTHERAPIST

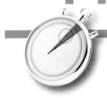

The innovative 3:21 Workout is the brainchild of Kusal Goonewardana, a highly qualified, trained and experienced sports physiotherapist, with more than 15 years of experience on his side. Let's take a deeper look into the logic and objectives of the 3:21 Workout as we know a bit more about the credentials of its enigmatic founder.

THE CREDENTIALS

Kusal Goonewardena is an Australian-based Sports Physiotherapist for elite athletes and the Head of Sports Medicine, University of Melbourne, since the year 2008. A PhD candidate in Sports Performance Enhancement in Melbourne, Goonewardena has a rich experience of more than 15 years of working in the high pressure sports medicine profession.

He renders his expert services for the Melbourne University Elite Athlete Unit, which comprises of 24 of the Melbourne's best athletes. A majority of these sportspeople go on to compete in the Summer Olympics, Winter Olympics, along with the other National Championships. In fact, Goonewardena has the distinction of looking after all the elite athletes who represent Australia from the University of Melbourne in any of these events.

His meritorious professional achievements have their base in a sound academic background. Following his interest in the field of sports medicine, Kusal Goonewardena did his Bachelor in Physiotherapy at the University of Melbourne, only to be followed by a Masters in Sports Physiotherapy from Latrobe University. His book, *Rid Your Back Pain in 21 Days or Less*, released in 2010 received a remarkable response and got him world-wide acclaim.

As a major measure of his illustrious achievements, Kusal Goonewardena is also the founder of the Vigor Sports Medicine Clinic chain in Melbourne, Australia. The clinics are the biggest and most comprehensive centers of their kind in their respective regions. The chains of clinics are also the only orthopedic teaching schools that train overseas qualified physiotherapists in Australia. Apart for the long lineage of athletes, Goonewardena has actually helped and trained 1000's of physiotherapists to excel in the field of sports physiotherapy.

Here, we've listed some of the most renowned and successful athletes who've trained under him:

✓ **Katya Crema**
  Winter Olympian and Ski Cross Champion

✓ **Christian Williams**
  Australian National Archer

✓ **Jeff Tho**
  Commonwealth Games badminton semi-finalist

✓ **Luke Chong**
  Oceania badminton champion

✓ **Phoebe Stanley**
  Australian Olympic Rower

✓ **Freddy Ovett**
  Australian Cyclist/Triathlete

✓ **Lachlan Norris**
  Australian Professional Cyclist and Motor Cross champion

✓ **Tom Swallow**
  Australian U-23 volleyball champion

✓ **Michelle Motteram**
  Victorian State Touch Rugby

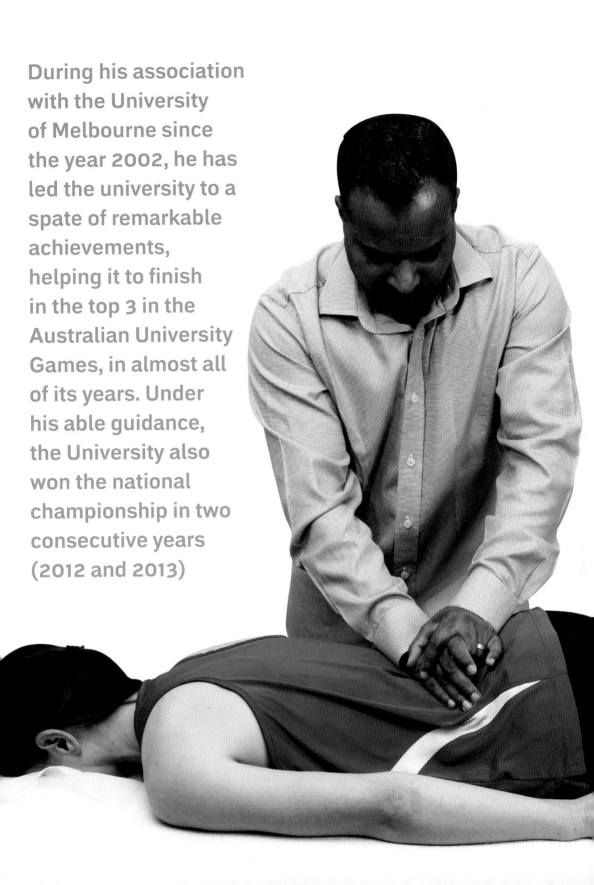

During his association with the University of Melbourne since the year 2002, he has led the university to a spate of remarkable achievements, helping it to finish in the top 3 in the Australian University Games, in almost all of its years. Under his able guidance, the University also won the national championship in two consecutive years (2012 and 2013)

Before we go on to see how the elite physiotherapist actually goes about his successful work plans, let's take a very quick look at some of the noteworthy achievements under his able guidance:

✓ More than 400 athletes compete under Australian University Games under his guidance every year.

✓ The University athletes have always finished in the top 5 since 2008, since Goonewardena took on the charge of the Sports Medicine.

✓ The University also won the overall National Championship for two executive years in 2012 and 2013.

THE 10 KEY FOCUS AREAS

Kusal Goonewardena, with his own unique vision about sports medicine and physiotherapy, has conducted more than 50,000 treatments during his entire career that spans well over a decade. Travelling all over the world to deliver his highly effective and successful workshops, he has always striven to maximize the potential of his athletes. He also organizes a series of webinars to be able to reach to a wider audience.

Training over 400 athletes every year, Goonewardena focuses on special skills and areas of performance that need to be polished to help the sportspersons excel.

Apart for the long lineage of athletes, Goonewardena has actually helped and trained 1000's of physiotherapists to excel in the field of sports physiotherapy.

Here's a list out of what all does Kusal strive to achieve with his clients and what are his key focus areas:

1 Strives to push the level of performance to the highest point, often taking the athlete from a mere 30% to a whopping 80% in as less as 21 days

2 Advising the athletes on high-power, result-oriented workouts within minimum time

3 Helps athletes to recover from their injuries in the shortest possible duration

4 Identifies their core strengths and trains athletes to perform to their maximum capacity during their event

5 Addresses groups and workshops on a regular basis so that a maximum number of sportspersons and specialists can benefit from his expertise

6 Teaching the athletes suitable self-body analysis before seeing a physiotherapist

7 Teaching sports specific mediation, a 3000 years old technique aimed at improving overall performance

8 Teaching the art of handling competition and performance pressure to the sportspersons

9 Training the sportspersons to develop a holistic approach towards training and preparation

10 3:21 - The New Age Workout

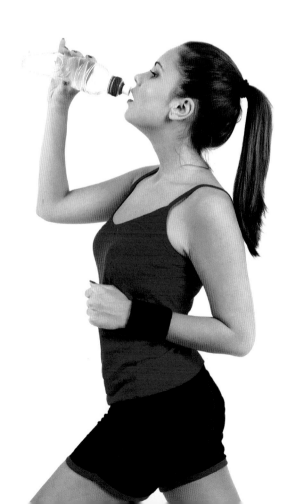

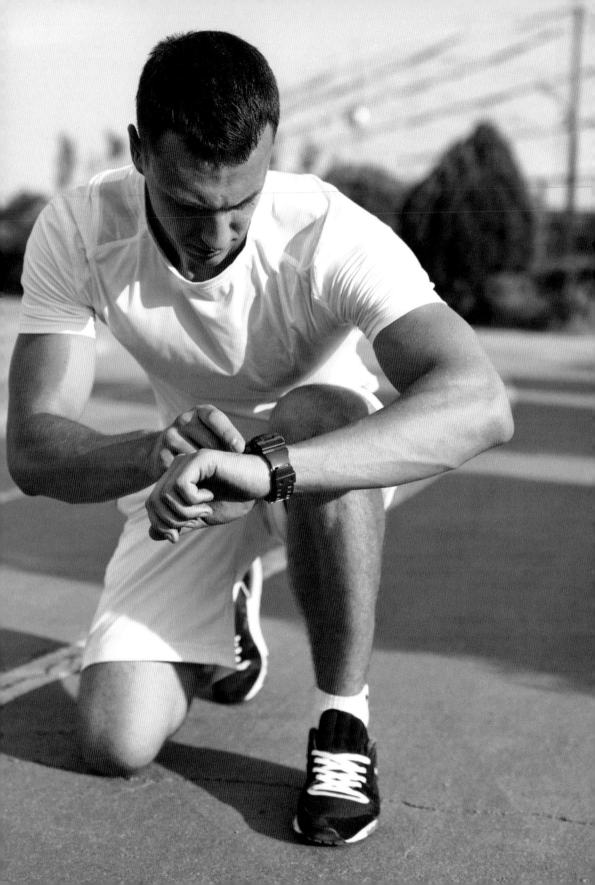

3:21 – THE NEW AGE WORKOUT

In the previous section, we read all about how short duration, high intensity interval training has definitely come to stay as the new age fitness solution.

Great in variety, quicker to do and with results amazingly visible, the HIIT has made concrete inroads into our self-management schedules.

In this section of the book, we will tell you about one of the most successful and target-oriented HIIT schedules, the 3:21 routine. A fitness routine so compact, it can easily fit into the tightest compartments of your busy routine. With results obvious to you as promised, the 3:21 brings to you all the glory of a premium HIIT routine, while carefully omitting the few drawbacks of this new age workout.

Read on as we give you a detailed account of the amazing 3:21 workout, what it really means, how to carry out, the pros and cons and everything else that you might want to know about the workout.

DEFINING 3:21

HIIT comes into its best form when specific, tailor-made sub-modules are scheduled into water-tight compartments in the shortest duration possible.

The 3:21 is one of the best templates of HIIT available today.

The 3:21 is an innovative, result-oriented HIIT template, designed as a combination of the some of the most crucial and important fitness regimens.

WHY 3:21 – CHALLENGES AND OBJECTIVES

The workout derives its name from the duration and time format of the exercises. The 3:21 workout basically includes 6 high-intensity workouts of 30 seconds each, to be done for 3 minutes every day, for a total of 21 days.

The workout has been especially designed for professionals who face a serious time crunch but intend to stay at the peak of their fitness level.

Let's move on to understand the structure and time devotion in detail.

During his illustrious years at the University and also through his interaction with elite athletes worldwide, Kusal Goonewardena was able to identify a few core challenges that almost all of the sportspersons faced today.

Keeping these problems and challenges in view, he designed the path-breaking 3:21 program, in order to fulfill the following critical objectives. Here, we've listed out the most problematic zones faced by the modern sportspersons and also how Goonewardena's new program promises to address each one of them.

1 THE TIME CRUNCH

The Challenge

Nowadays, most of the sportspersons multi-task between their jobs, education and sports. Working part time or even full time or studying to get their academic credentials updated, they often find themselves strapped for time for rigorous workouts, traditionally required to maintain their fitness levels. Moreover, they often have hectic travel schedules that don't allow long spans of stead-state exercises. Meanwhile, the professional athletes are already bound with task of competitions and events, which often leaves them with very less time for long workouts.

The 3:21 Advantage

As the basic principle suggests, this workout only takes 3 minutes every day to complete. Packed with 6 mini modules of just 30 seconds each, the program offers maximum advantage in the minimum amount of time.

2 PRONE TO LOSS OF FOCUS

With such myriad forms of tasks to finish, today's sportspersons can quite easily lose focus on fitness. Unlike earlier days, a sportsperson is not only required to stay fit, but also perform other tasks like participate in social events, travel extensively and even study further to improve their academic records.

The 3:21 advantage

The workouts of the 3:21 program are highly focused and result oriented. They target each of the essential aspects of the required fitness levels. All that is required is a complete focus on the activities at hand for those 3 minutes and the athlete stands no chance of loss of focus.

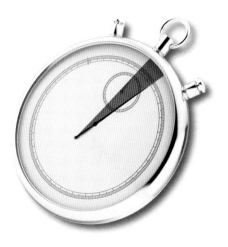

3 IMBALANCED BENEFITS

Most of the conventional workouts are laden with the risk of an imbalanced impact on the body all over. It often happens that the entire benefit of the exercises is either borne by the legs, abdomen or the bust area. In the absence of proper guidance and supervision, it often becomes difficult to do a workout that has a balanced impact for all aspects of the body.

The 3:21 advantage

One of the biggest facts about the 3:21 program is its ability to target multiple groups of muscles at one time. Each of its 6 workouts is designed to target different muscle groups and hence offer overall benefit as against lop-sided benefits of the conventional workouts. For instance, the pushups and squat jumps bring into work both legs and arms muscles in an equal measure apart from aiming to tone the abdominal area as well.

4 HIGH SCOPE OF INJURIES

The Challenge

A huge proportion of professional sportsperson are likely to lose out on a lot of opportunities due to repetitive injuries, especially during their workouts. Being highly prone to injury, there fitness goals are easily marred. Since, it takes some time before they can recover, they are often forced to miss out on major events.

The 3:21 advantage

The 3:21 program helps you conduct your workouts with the minimal scope of injuries. Being professionally designed, it doesn't exert your ligaments or muscles in an undesirable manner, thereby avoiding any major injuries.

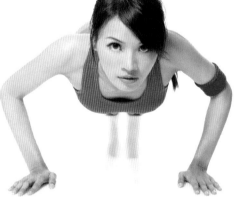

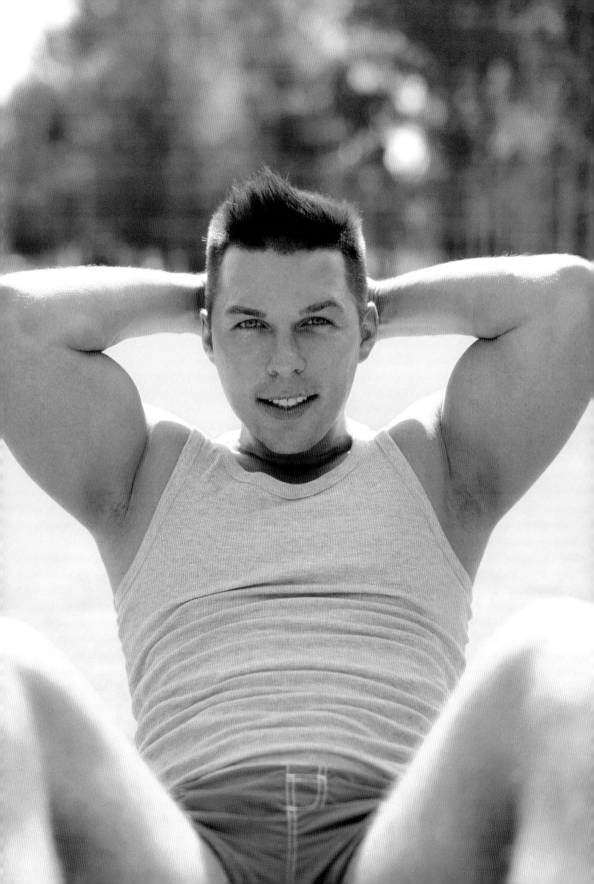

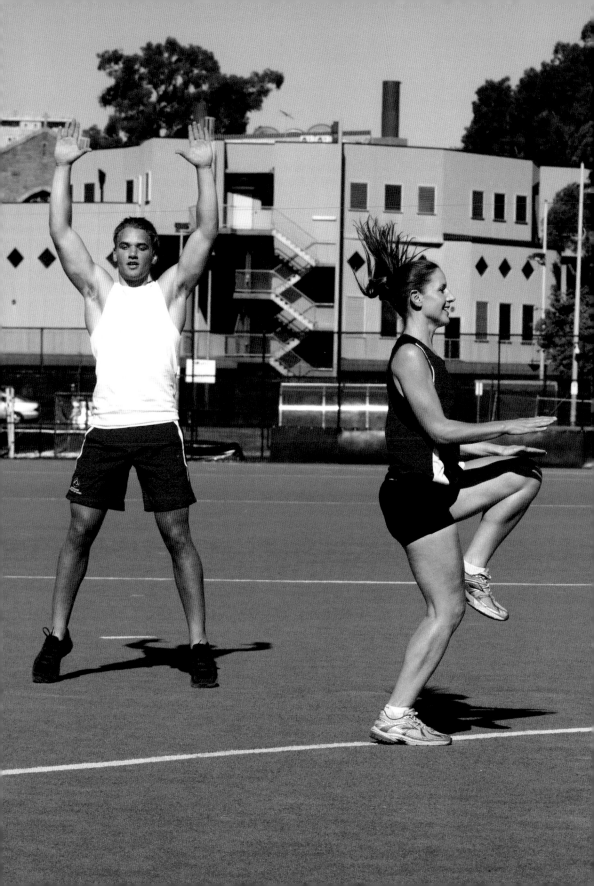

5 LOSS OF INTEREST

The Challenge
Steady state exercises often bring with them the risk of being monotonous. It is very common for sportspersons to lose interest in long and tedious exercises. With heavy exertion and minimal results visible in long-term, quite a few of those who exercise tend to drop in halfway.

The 3:21 advantage
The 3:21 program conquers this challenge by offering a dynamic sequence of workouts. The modules that make up this program offer a great variety and prevent any monotony creeping into the fitness regimen.

6 NEED FOR EQUIPMENT, STRUCTURE AND SPACE

The Challenge
One would normally exercise in routine within a specific duration at home or the gym and using specific equipment. Moreover, the workout requires space and also an ambience to be carried out. This can often act as a deterrent, especially for those who don't have a fixed routine or travel often.

The 3:21 advantage
The 3:21 Workout can be done anywhere, without any equipment and above all at any time of the day. The usual constraints of space and gymnasium membership are not relevant to the 3:21 Workout at all. In fact, the 3:21 Workout is not even marred by any financial constraint as it is almost a free-of-cost workout.

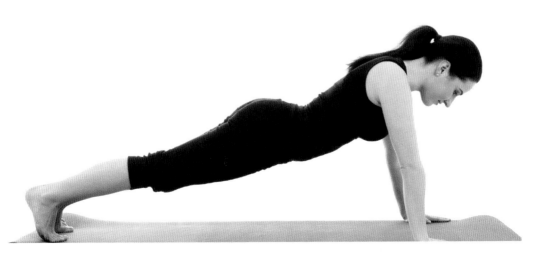

THE LOGIC OF 85%

Before we go on to understand the key underlying logic of the 3:21 Workout, let's take a closer look at the actual format of a conventional, steady-state exercise.

The traditional form of exercise has three conspicuous features that define the kind of workouts we do, which are:

✓ **Use of equipment**

✓ **Loss of muscle and fat**

✓ **Exercising within the specific aerobic zone**

However, the 3:21 Workout redefines each of these features and gives an all-new meaning to fitness.

As per the modules of this program, we are not required to use any equipment. The athletes are typically required to use their own body weight to exercise and push themselves beyond their typical aerobic zone.

The basic principle of the 3:21 Workout plan lies in pushing yourself to as much as the level of 85% of your capacity. The level is defined as such because as per experts, we can push up to the level of 85% without actually causing any major injury or strain to the ligaments. Moreover, you are only required to push yourself to 85% for very short bursts of time .i.e. for 3 minutes each only.

THE FOUNDER'S VISION

According to Kusal Goonewardena, the founder of the 3:21 Workout, this logic helps in a lot of ways, some of which include:

✓ **Athletes only use their own body weight to push themselves to the specified 85%, thereby eliminating the need of any additional equipment or resources.**

✓ **Since the exercise spurts are only of 3 minutes and you control the intensity, the risk of injury is at its minimum.**

DURATION AND STRUCTURE

3:21 Workout is a structured, 6-part fitness routine typically carried out in capsules of 3 minutes every day.

It is so structured to enable maximum utilization of the exercise ability of the athlete, with minimum injury and within the shortest span of time.

The basic structure of the 3:21 Workout comprises of 6 modules of 30 seconds each, packed into a combined session of 3 minutes. This 3-minute session is to be done for 21 days at a stretch, as per the pattern laid out.

Each of the modules has been selected to solve particular fitness issues.

In the words of the founder Kusal Goonewardana,

"While there are many variations of the high-intensity workout, I chose the exercises to target specific parts of the body and because anyone can do them."

Goonewardana points out that the exercises are primarily meant to strengthen the arms and leg strength and help condition the body, preparing it for exercise or other forms of higher intensity exercises and sports in the future.

Before we understand the exact structure, first let's know more about what these workouts focus on.

The entire 3:21 workout has three main fitness areas as its main target points, which include:

✓ **Upper body strengthening and conditioning**

✓ **Lower body strengthening and conditioning**

✓ **Core control and conditioning**

Each of the above objectives is achieved by a separate set of workouts. The instructor makes a judgment based on the athlete's body condition about the particular set to be followed. As described earlier, the athlete then does the decided set of exercises for a continuous span of 3 minutes.

Here, we've listed all the workouts that are to be done for each of the above 3 fitness objectives.

✓ Shadow boxing

✓ Push ups

✓ Squat jumps

✓ High knee running, on the spot

✓ Star jumps

✓ Sit ups

The basic structure of the 3:21 Workout comprises of 6 modules of 30 seconds each, packed into a combined session of 3 minutes. This 3-minute session is to be done for 21 days at a stretch, as per the pattern laid out.

3 Core Fitness Objectives

UPPER BODY STRENGTH/CONDITIONING

Shadow boxing

Push ups

LOWER BODY STRENGTH/CONDITIONING

Squat jumps

High knee running, on the spot

CORE CONTROL AND CONDITIONING

Star jumps

Sit ups

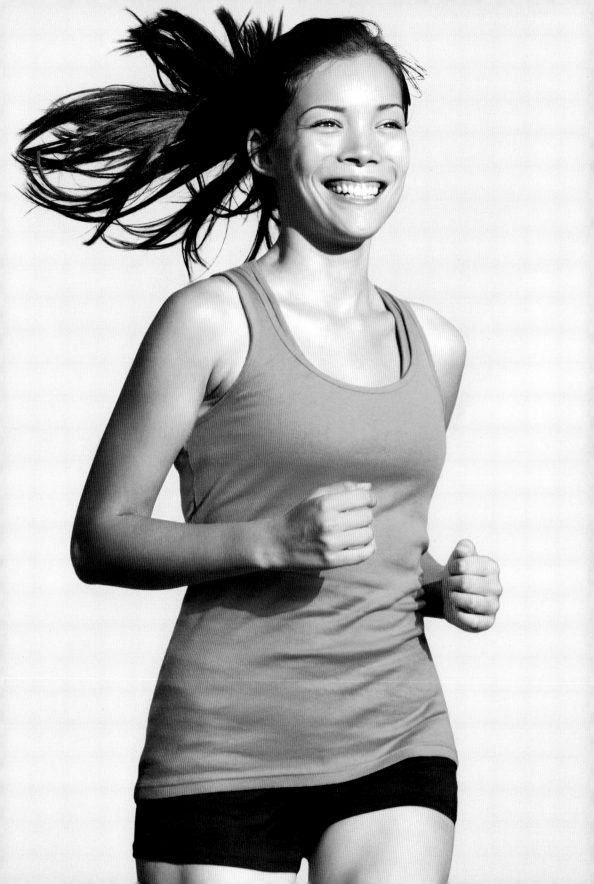

3:21– 5 QUESTIONS YOU MUSK ASK

It sounds like a miracle; a power-packed, result-oriented workout package that promises to show so many benefits, it is natural for suspicions to arise. In this section, we've listed five such important frequently asked questions which will quell all your doubts about the 3:21 program.

1 WHY 21 DAYS

Well, there's an indeed an interesting tale behind it! It was way back in the 1950s when the plastic surgeon Maxwell Maltz noticed a weird pattern in his patterns. Maltz noticed that most of his patients would take something like 21 days to get adjusted to their new look, such as a new nose, a re-defined lip and so on.

"These, and many other commonly observed phenomena tend to show that it requires a minimum of about 21 days for an old mental image to dissolve and a new one to jell.", observed Maltz.

In specific relevance to the 3:21 program, the modules are designed as such that it takes them around 21 days to begin showing an impact. According to the founder of the program, Kusal Goonewardena, after a period of 21 days, the body gets so accustomed to the workout, that there is innate desire to do the same.

2 WHY ONLY 3 MINUTES

Here, the answer lies in the nature of the workouts. The 3:21 program is based on the logic that high intensity, short duration workouts have a different and most of the times, a stronger impact on the body than the conventional steady-state, low intensity exercises such walking or simple jogging.

3 WHY HIGH INTENSITY

Here, the answer again lies in the underlying logic of the 3:21 program. Each of the modules of the program requires pushing yourself to at least 80% of your capacity. This is to ensure that the desired effect takes place on the rate of calories being burnt, your heart rate, impact on the muscles and so on.

4 CAN EVERYONE DO IT?

Well, not everyone. Though the modules in the 3:21 program are fairly easy to do, yet you do require a certain degree of fitness to take up the same. Since some of the workouts require steps with heavy exertion, you might end up hurting yourself if you are absolutely a beginner to exercise.

5 WHEN WILL I SEE THE RESULTS?

You will start feel energetic and healthier in as early as 1 week. However, for the real results of the 3:21 program to be visible, you will have to give the workout at least 21 days to the minimum. Refer to the earlier section of this part to know more about the underlying logic of the 21 days duration and why your body takes at least this much of time to show the results.

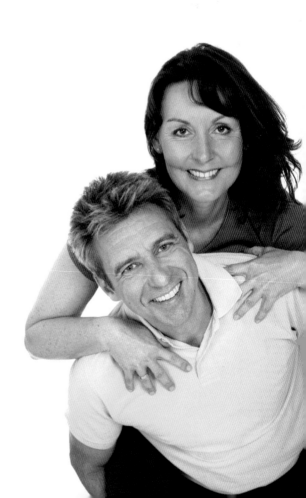

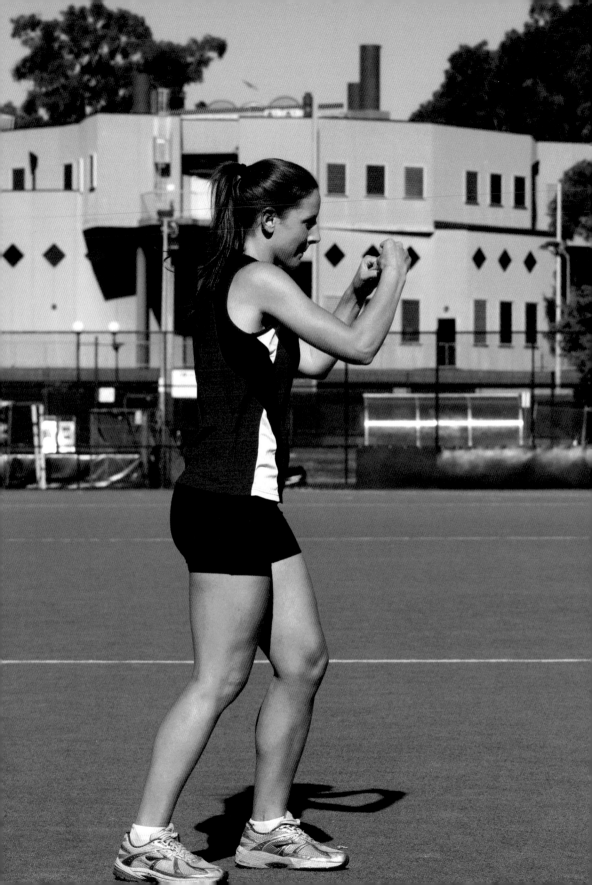

THE 6 WORKOUTS

In this section, we've explained each of the six workouts in detail, with guidelines on how to do the workout in the correct manner in order to get the best of results.

1 SHADOW BOXING

This particular workout is the first exercise when it comes to Upper Body Strength and Conditioning.

Let's begin by understanding more about the workout, its benefits and the right way to carry it out.

ABOUT SHADOW BOXING

Shadow Boxing is traditionally considered to be one of the oldest, most effective and versatile exercises that help the sportsperson in improving all aspects of fighting ability.

As per its definition, Shadow Boxing is a technique in which the boxer or fighter moves around swiftly in the ring, throwing punches in the air, as if fighting an invisible opponent. As the name suggests, shadow boxing prompts the athlete to box with a shadow. It is known to sharpen the athlete's fighting techniques and condition their muscles.

The workout is so called because in shadow boxing, the boxers usually pretend to box with their shadow on a wall or with a mirror in front of them.

SHADOW BOXING AND 3:21 WORKOUT

Shadow boxing is one of the most relevant and important aspects of the Upper Body Conditioning and Strengthening module of the 3:21 workout. To begin with, it requires absolutely no equipment or infrastructure. Secondly, shadow boxing improves your reflexes and pace of workout as it involves very quick responses to an imaginary opponent. It also improves your focus and concentration, thereby increasing your overall output from the workout. In fact, shadow boxing is known to be helpful for increasing your overall strength, endurance, speed and stamina.

One of the other key benefits of shadow boxing is that it doesn't tire you out. It also gets your muscles into a systematic rhythm of movement, which will help you while performing other parts of the 3:21 workout.

As a workout, some of the most important benefits of shadow boxing include:

✓ **To help in warming up the muscles, joints and ligaments for further workouts**

✓ **To improve the footwork and legwork of the athlete**

✓ **To develop and improve the coordination amongst muscles and joints**

✓ **To improve the athlete's visualization techniques**

✓ **To improve cardio and conditioning**

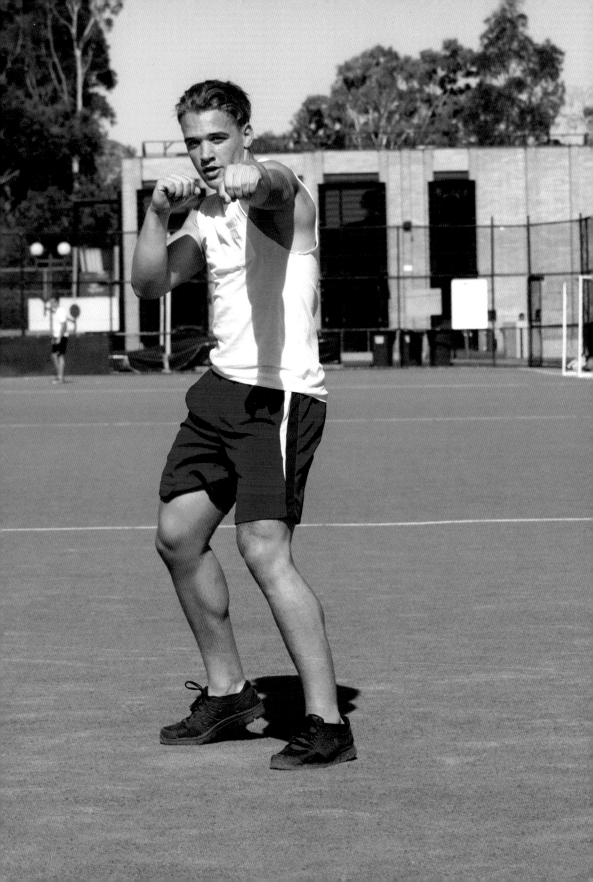

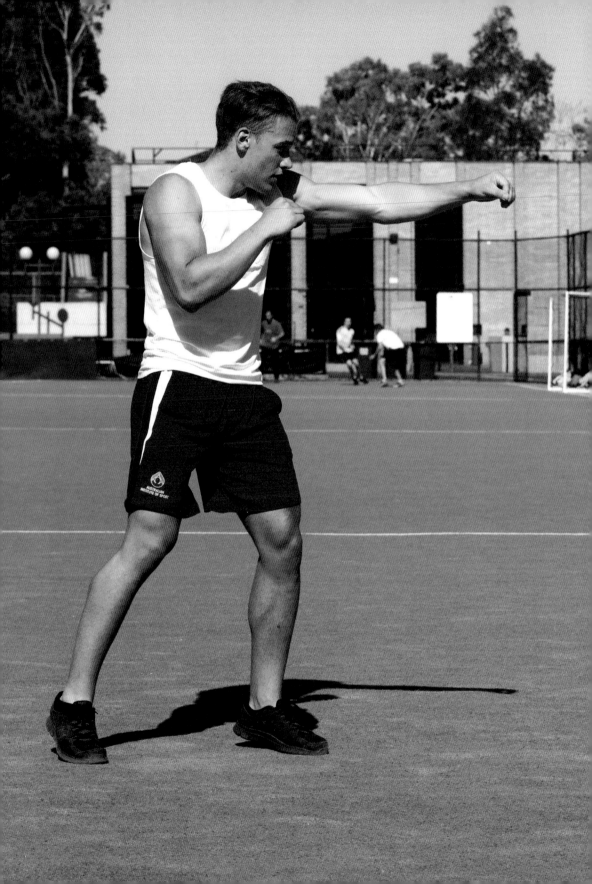

HOW TO DO SHADOW BOXING – THE 3 KEY WAYS

There are a huge number of ways in which you can do shadow boxing. In this section, we've furnished brief details of 3 key shadow boxing drills that you can use.

1 MOVEMENT SHADOWBOXING

In this form of shadow boxing, you will start by not throwing any punches and concentrating on your movement instead. All you need to do is to just move forwards, backwards, pivot, hop and pendulum step. This will help you in developing agility and coordination amongst your bodily movements.

2 PIVOT/T FRAME SHADOWBOXING

This pattern involves basic shadow boxing, with key focus on maintaining the T-frame. You have to focus on keeping your shoulders above your knees and pivoting in the right manner as you throw your punches.

3 SPEED SHADOW BOXING

This particular method increases the athlete's speed and time of response. Making sure that the punches are technically correct, the sportsman is just required to throw as much punches as possible in a limited, pre-decided span of time. This particular pattern gives the best result when there are 2 or more people doing it, since it increases the level of competitiveness and hence improves performance.

2 PUSH UPS

Pushups are traditionally considered to be one of the most effective and convenient forms of exercises to do. A typical workout that uses the athlete's body weight along with force of gravity to bring the desired results, pushups can be done by athletes of all levels, whether amateurs or professionals. Before we go on to understand the proper techniques of doing various types of push-ups, first let's understand more about the workout and how it is relevant to the 3:21 regimen.

The most important fact about pushups that make them such an important workout is that it is much a resistance exercise as it is a strength-building workout.

ABOUT PUSH-UPS

An integral part of the upper body strength and conditioning regimen, pushups work on almost each of your muscle between your shoulders and toes.

The most important fact of pushups that make them such an important workout is that it is as much a resistance exercise as it is a strength-building workout. It works on multiple body muscles and joints at the same time, hence bringing you a string of benefits.

In the section that follows, we've listed some of the most important benefits of doing the push-ups as a part of the 3:21 workout.

PUSHUPS AND 3:21 WORKOUT – THE BENEFITS

Given the simplicity of pushups, they form a perfect part of the 3:21 workout. The relevance of pushups to the 3:21 workout is especially high in the light of the effective results and the minimum time taken to do the exercise.

Here, we've listed out some of the most important benefits of the workout, in specific relevance to the 3:21 regimen.

✓ **Overall strengthening**
Pushups are known to be the most effective form of workouts for building up bodily strength. This workout works on all the muscles in the upper body and builds strengths in forearms, chest and shoulders.

✓ **Strengthens the core**
This particular part of the 3:21 Workout makes an impact on the core by stabilizing the abdominals and back. The force exerted during the push works on these muscles in a considerable way.

✓ **Enhances metabolic rate**
Since push-ups use a lot of muscles at the same time, including the ones in your legs. This, in turn implies that your heart has to work harder to pump the blood to your muscles, causing an increase in the breathing rate. Your metabolic rate gets affected since your body works to recover even after the workout is over, which means that more energy in burnt.

✓ **Convenient and feasible**
A push-up requires no equipment, minimal space and takes very less time. All of these factors are highly important and crucial in any workout which is done as a part of the 3:21 Workout.

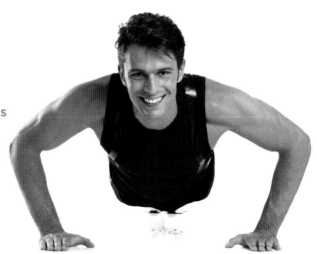

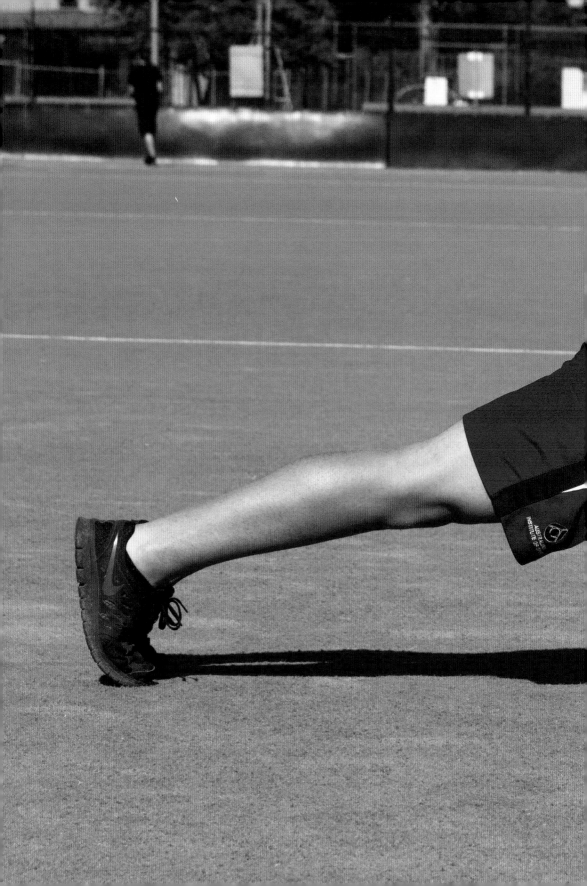

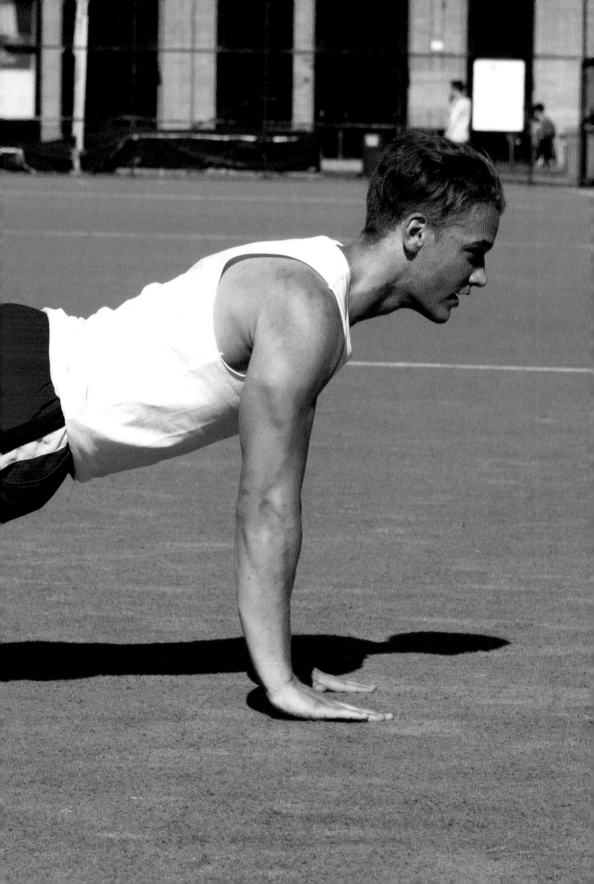

PUSH UPS – THE RIGHT METHOD

Pushups have a huge series of variations and the workout can be performed in a lot of different ways. In this section, we've demonstrated the right way to do the pushups in a systematic and step-wise manner.

STEPS

1 Lie down on the floor, face down, with your hands a bit wider than your shoulders

2 Contract your core and tighten your abs slightly by pulling your belly button inwards towards your spine

3 Lift up your body, balancing on your toes and hands

4 Ensure that your body remains straight, without sagging in the middle or arching your back

5 Slowly inhale as you straighten your elbows and raise your body, halting as your elbows are straightened without locking

6 Exhale and lower yourself to the start position

7 Do not straighten your elbows fully, keeping them slightly bent

The relevance of pushups to the 3:21 workout is especially high in the light of the effective results and the minimum time taken to do the exercise.

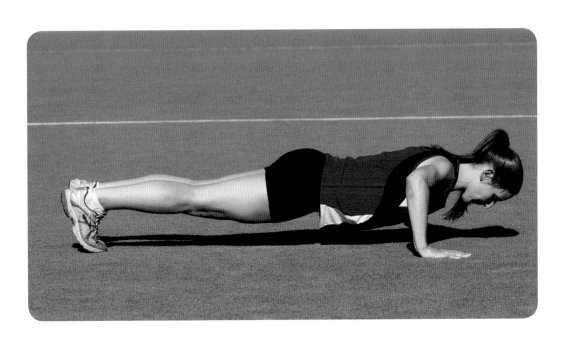

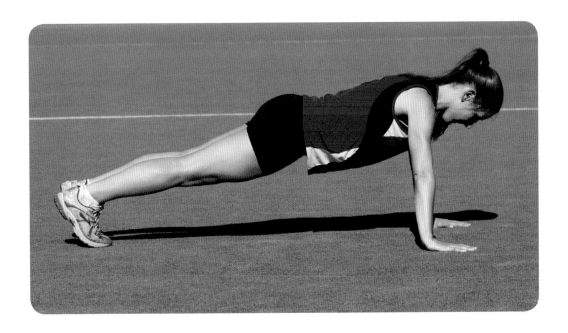

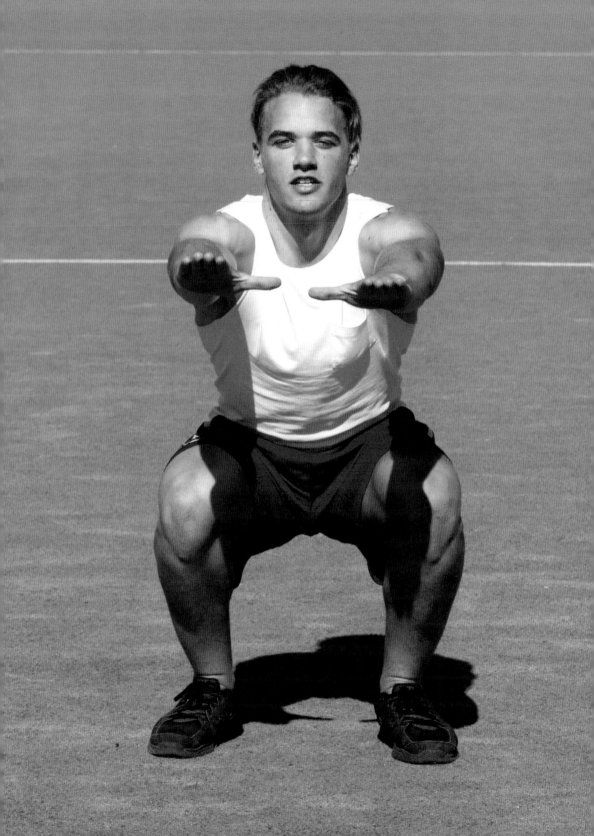

3 SQUAT JUMPS

A squat jump is basically a combination workout that brings together the movements of a squatting position and jump. Though initially perceived as a leg exercise, recent research has shown squat jumps to be an equally effective exercise for muscle building and fat loss throughout the body. Let's read a bit more about the squat jumps before we go on to understand its relevance to the 3:21 workout.

ABOUT JUMP SQUATS

A jump squat is an extensive full-body workout for the legs and the core. It aims to improve the athlete's explosive strength by pushing him to jump out of the squat position. Considered as a full body workout, the squat jumps work extensively on the legs and midsection, including the gluteus maximum, hamstrings, abdominals, carves and quadriceps.

3:21 AND BENEFITS

Squat jumps, as a part of the lower body strengthening or conditioning portion of the 3:21 Workout bring along a series of benefits to the athletes and sportsmen. Some of the most important benefits include:

✓ Squat jump is essentially a functional exercise. This implies it helps you to perform your daily routine activities also easily as against the other usual workouts that are limited to the gym. Being able to squat and get up comfortably helps you to perform a lot of activities in your day with ease

✓ The most important benefit of squat jumps lies in their ability to build the legs muscles and create an anabolic environment, which encourages build up of muscles throughout the body

✓ The workout requires no equipment, less space and minimal time. All of these are essential pre-requisites of the 3:21 Workout

✓ Squat jumps are known to be very effective in toning your gluteals and legs.

✓ It helps in maintaining the mobility in the sportspersons as they age

✓ It helps in enhancing the upper body strength owing to the large amounts of growth hormone and testosterone released through squatting

✓ It enhances vertical jump in basketball and also explosiveness in sports like football

✓ As another unconventional benefit, squat jumps are good for the waste removal system of your body since it improves the pumping of body fluids and aids in waste removal

✓ The strengthened and toned muscles that occur as a result of the squat jumps help in reducing the rate of injuries to the muscles. The increased flexibility in the muscles also helps in lowering the injury rate.

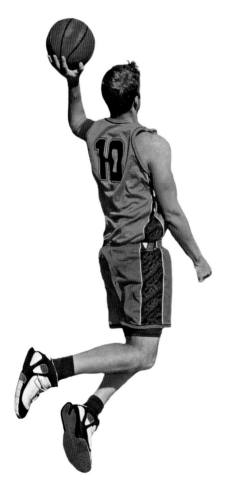

STEPS

1 Stand straight, with your legs shoulder width apart

2 Your toes should be pointing outwards

3 If you are a beginner, keep your arms parallel to your body. If you can keep your balance, then place your hands on your head

4 Bend and sit back like you are sitting on a bench or a chair

5 Break at the hips before you bend your knees

6 Keeping your back straight, lower yourself down until your thighs are parallel to the floor

7 Go as further down as you can

8 Once you are at the bottom, jump up as high as you can

9 Keep your knees bent as you jump up

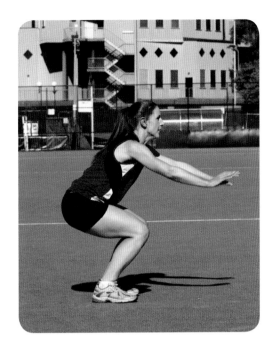

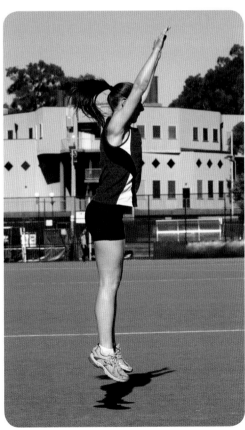

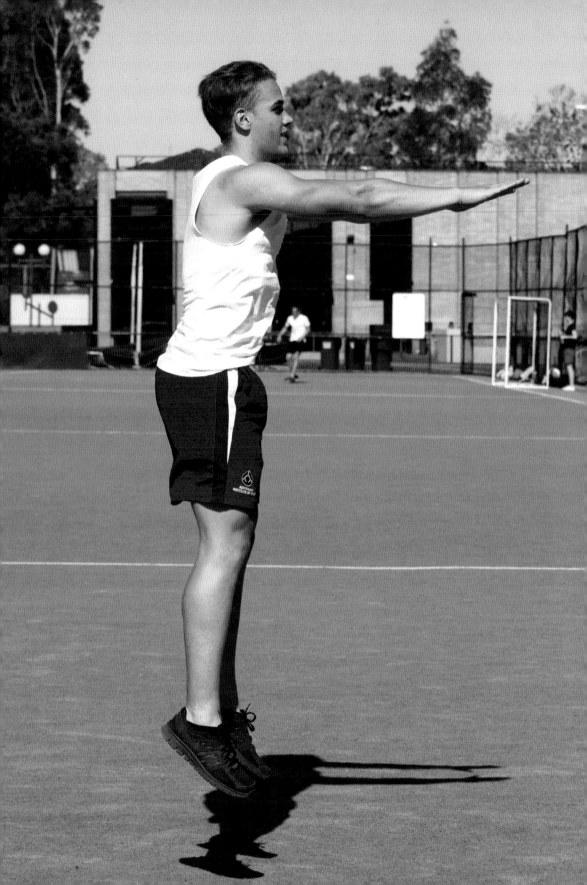

POINTS TO REMEMBER

Certain points need to be kept in mind while performing the squat jumps. Here, we've listed some of the most important guidelines:

✓ Weight should come down through your heels

✓ Feet should be kept only shoulder width apart

✓ Spine should be kept neutral

✓ Ensure that the knees don't go any further than the toes

✓ When you jump up, aim for the height, aim to 'grow tall'

✓ If you pause between jumps, the amount of stored elasticity reduces, making the workout harder

Did you know...

It is indeed amazing that as per research, squat jumps, when done properly, can actually trigger the release of the human growth hormone in the body, which is in tune, very crucial for muscle growth.

As another very non-conventional benefit, squat jumps are good for the waste removal system of your body since it improves the pumping of body fluids and aids in waste removal

4 HIGH KNEE RUNNING (ON THE SPOT)

High knee running is one of the many types of running drills that can be performed by athletes and sports persons to increase their strength and speed. It is the second module as a part of the lower body strength and conditioning objective of the 3:21 Workout.

Various types of running drill can be performed to add on to your daily workouts. The 3:21 Workout incorporates on-the-spot high knee running into its regimen for a series of reasons.

Let's understand more about this particular workout before we understand its benefits and specific relevance to the 3:21 program.

ABOUT HIGH KNEE RUNNING

Also known as running-in place, high knee running is widely regarded as an excellent warm up routine and also a great strength building exercise. The second part of the lower body strengthening and conditioning portion of the 3:21 program, on-the-spot high knee running builds your endurance levels, stamina and also the speed.

THE BENEFITS

Experts point out at a series of benefits of the high knee running workout, which makes it especially relevant to the basic principle of the 3:21 program.

Some of the key benefits are:

✓ **The workout has multiple effects on various bodily functions. It strengthens the lungs and improves the circulatory and respiratory system.**

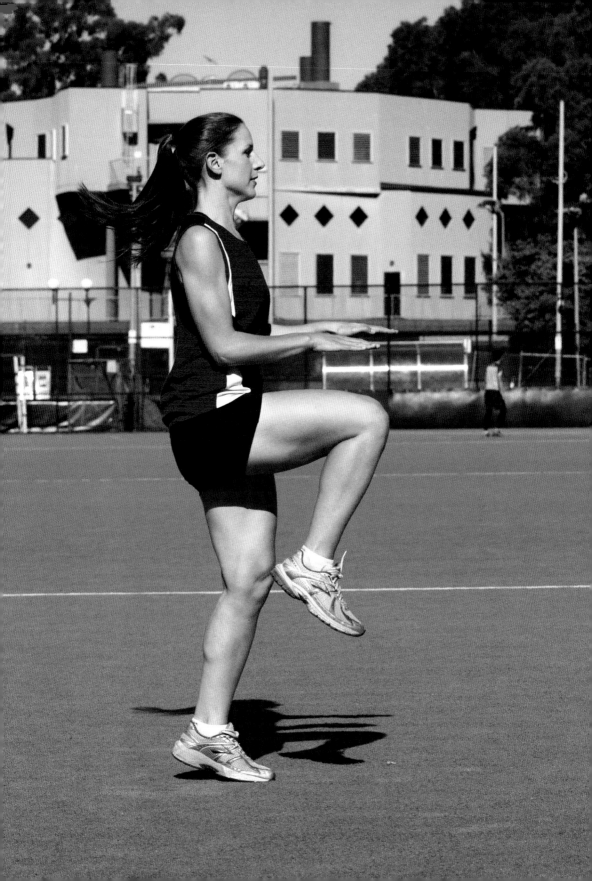

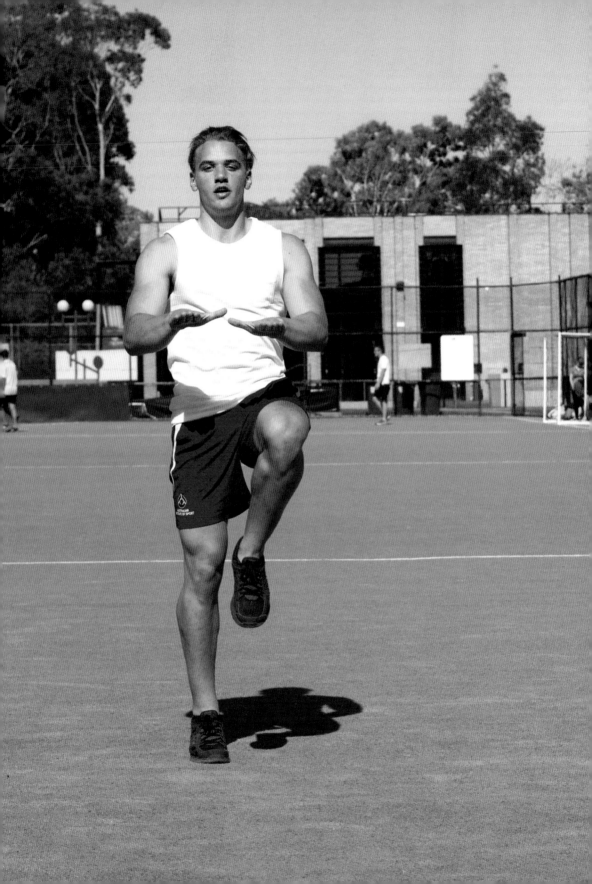

✓ As with all modules of the 3:21 program, on the spot high knee running is convenient and economical. It doesn't need any equipment or even much of space.

✓ It increases your heart rate and burns calories at a stable pace.

✓ It gives a good workout to your thighs, hips, calf and gluteal muscles.

✓ It also works out your quadriceps and hamstring muscles, calf muscles.

✓ It enhances the level of oxygen intake for an improved cellular health.

✓ It tones your muscles in a highly effective manner

✓ It enhances your heart rate. It also helps in reducing the risks of osteoporosis, diabetes, high cholesterol and even some types of cancer.

✓ Owing to the high rate of calories being burnt, running in place can lead to effective weight loss.

STEPS

There are a series of different ways in which the high knee running can be done as a part of the 3:21 Workout. In this section, we've listed down the basic steps in a sequential manner:

1 Stand straight in an open place. Take a deep breath.

2 Start by slowly running, on the spot. Keep your shoulders relaxed and arms bent at the sides.

3 Increase your speed slowly.

4 Once your speed is fast enough, start pulling up your knees to the waist height.

5 Make sure to keep your shoulders pulled back and straight.

6 With each knee rise pat your knee with your hand.

POINTS TO REMEMBER

Although high knee running is a very helpful workout and works wonders for athletes, there are certain points that need to be kept in mind when doing this particular workout. Here, we've listed some of the most important precautions and point that need to be kept in mind while doing this particular workout as a part of the 3:21 Workout.

✓ Though it holds true for all other workout as well, but make sure you are wearing the right training shoes in this particular exercise to avoiding hurting your knees or feet.

✓ If you are new to this exercise, being by high knee marching instead of running, on the spot.

✓ Remember to lift only one knee at a time, straight and as high as possible.

✓ Make sure you breathe properly through the workout.

✓ Gradually try to increase the height of your knee as it comes up to your chest.

✓ Stay away from concrete and firm surfaces.

✓ Remember to stretch and warm up before the exercise and cool down properly once the exercise is over.

It enhances your heart rate. It also helps in reducing the risks of osteoporosis, diabetes, high cholesterol and even some types of cancer.

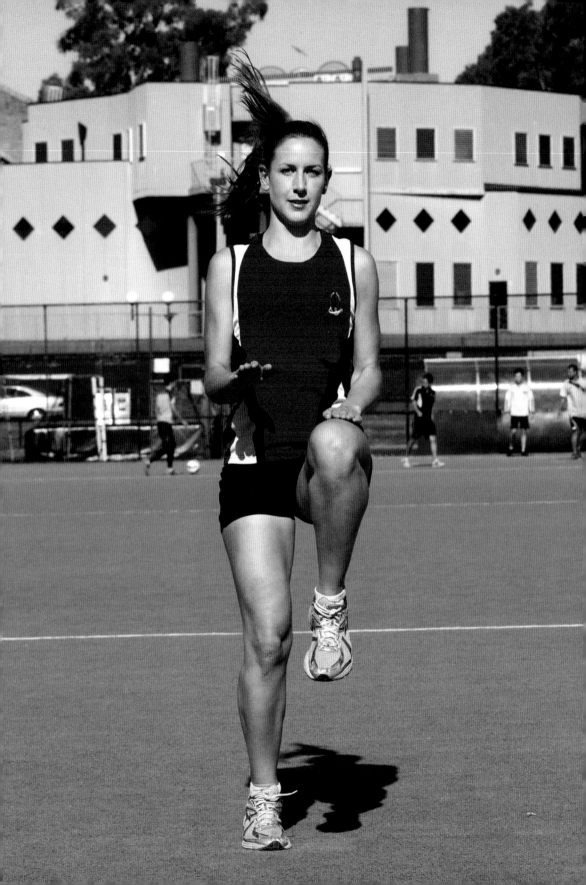

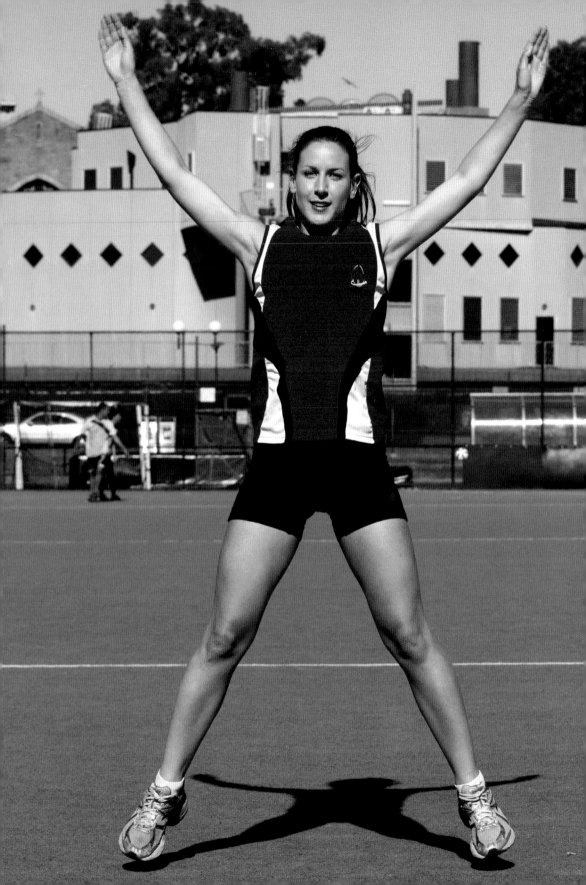

5 STAR JUMPS

The first part of the core control and conditioning, star jumps form an integral part of the 3:21 Workout. Also known as the Jumping Jacks in some parts of the world, this exercise involves rapid and high intensity jumps with heavy use of arms and legs. It has a special relevance with the 3:21 Workout owing to the high intensity of the workout.

Let's read a bit more on the star jumps, it's benefits and how it is an important part of the

ABOUT STAR JUMPS

Athletes can generally opt from one of the two types of star jumps, which are:

✓ Star Burst – In this type of star jumping, the jumping step is done in one quick movement.

✓ The 2-Step Star Burst – In this variation, the athlete basically lands with his feet out wide before he returns to the standing position.

Star jumps are effective in losing weight and excess fat mass, if done properly.

THE 3:21 WORKOUT AND STAR JUMPS

Star Jumps carry a vast range of benefits as a workout and also as a component of the 3:21 Workout. Some of the key benefits of star jumps, in specific relevance to the 3:21 Workout include:

✓ Foremost, star jumps are an excellent module for overall toning of the arms and legs muscles.

✓ They enhance overall cardiovascular fitness.

✓ They also target a wide range of muscles including the hamstrings, deltoids and glutes.

✓ This workout increases your heart rate and hence, increases the number of calories burnt.

✓ Star jumps are effective in losing weight and excess fat mass, if done properly.

✓ Due to its effect on the heart rate, star jumps also improve overall breathing manner in the individual.

STEPS

In this section, we've explained the proper series of steps in which the star burst variation of the star jumps can be carried out. Read on for a detailed description of the steps.

1 Stand straight with ample vacant space around you.

2 Bend your legs at the knees. Go down only a bit.

3 With a slight jerk, jump upwards and outwards.

4 As you do the above step, open your legs wide and move your arms out.

5 To check whether you are doing it right, create a star shape on the air.

6 The next step is the landing.

7 Bend your knees until your hands can touch the floor on both the sides.

8 Remember to keep your back straight.

9 Jump back again into the star shape.

10 Pause after 10 sets and repeat.

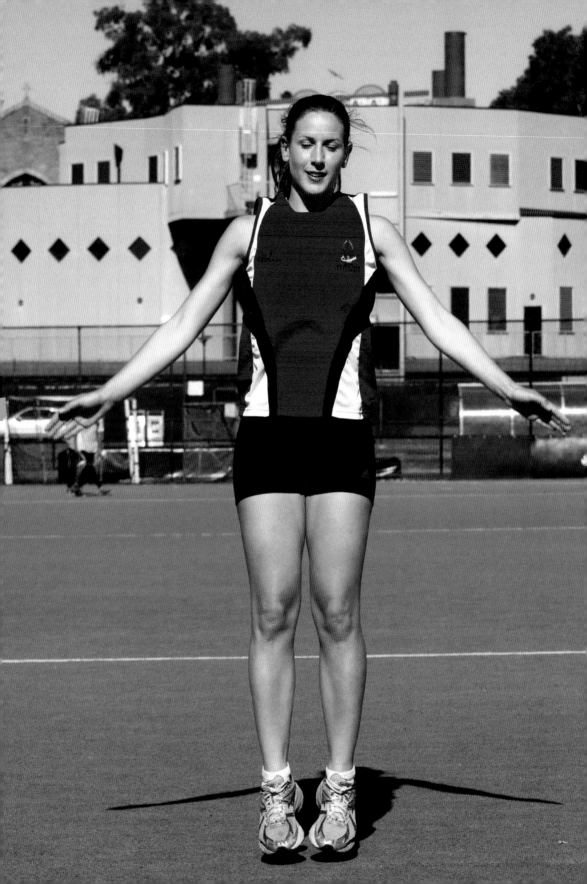

6 SIT UPS

Widely regarded as the most commonly performed abdominal exercise, sit ups can be done by individuals of all levels, provided they are done in the right manner. In this section, we will tell you all about this wonderful workout, how it is relevant to the 3:21 workout, steps to do it the right way and finally, some important points to remember. Let's begin by getting to know the workout more.

A sit up is basically an abdominal strength training workout that primarily targets the abdominal muscles.

ABOUT SIT UPS

A sit up is basically an abdominal strength training workout that primarily targets the abdominal muscles. Though commonly compared to crunches, sit ups offer a bigger range of motion and also target more muscles. In laymen terms, a sit up is an exercise in which the person lies on his back and uses his stomach muscles to raise the upper part of the body to a sitting position.

Sit ups are the second module adopted as a part of the core control and conditioning objective of the 3:21 Workout. From enhancing strength to toning up your body sit ups have an immense range of benefits especially in the context of the 3:21 Workout.

Here we've listed some of the most important benefits one can derive from this last workout of the 3:21 Workout.

THE BENEFITS

As a workout, sit ups bring along with them a host of benefits for the athletes, sportspersons and even laymen. In this section, we've listed out some of the most prominent benefits of this workout.

✓ They help in developing strong muscles.

✓ Sit ups tone the body in a lesser span of time than other exercises.

✓ The workout strengthens your 'external' core – the larger external abdominal muscles.

✓ They help in enhancing the stamina and endurance levels.

✓ Sit-ups work on the abdominal muscles extensively.

✓ The strength and flexibility obtained from this workout will also help you in your overall daily activities.

✓ This workout also develops overall stability and balance in your body as it works on your back, shoulder, abdomen, arms and hips, making them exert together.

✓ Owing to the well-toned abdominal muscles, your digestive system and posture also improve. This in turn, improves the flow of oxygen throughout the body.

✓ As one of the most important benefits, doing sit ups regularly can give you a fine physique and figure, with a muscular and lean appearance.

✓ As with all other workouts the 3:21 Workout, sit-ups do not require any formal equipment or a large open space.

The workout strengthens your 'external' core – the larger external abdominal muscles.

STEPS

As with most of the other workouts, sit ups also have a series of variations and can be done many different ways and patterns. In this section, we've listed out the standard steps for simple sit-ups. You can make changes to the level of intensity and duration gradually if you feel the need.

Follow these steps to perform sit ups with the right technique.

1 Lie down straight on the floor, with your feet under something to hold them back. You can also have a partner hold your feet for the purpose.

2 Bend your legs at the knees.

3 Get into the starting position. Place your hands behind your head, locking them by clasping your fingers or crossing them over your chest.

4 Look ahead and keep your chin slightly away from your chest. Make sure your neck is in a relaxed position.

5 Breathe in slowly.

6 Slowly lift your shoulders, head and neck.

7 Keep your lower back in contact with the floor.

8 Lift your shoulder away from the ground till your shoulder blades lift off the ground.

9 Exhale and Slowly return to the starting position.

As one of the most important benefits, doing sit ups regularly can give you a fine physique and figure, with a muscular and lean appearance.

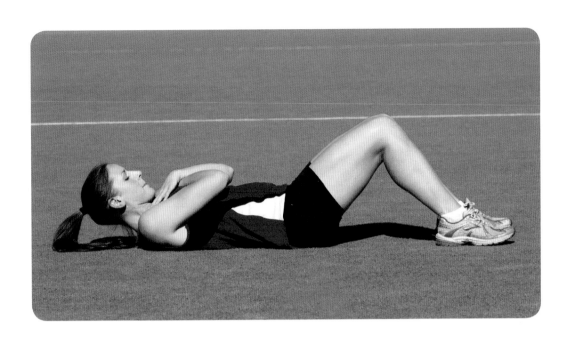

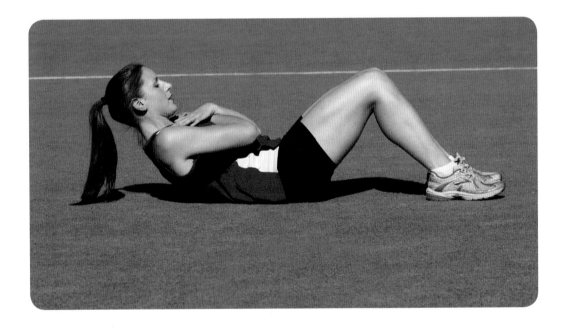

POINTS TO REMEMBER

Sit ups are undoubtedly one of the most effective workouts as a part of the 3:21 program. However, the workout is laden with some risks which require the athlete to keep a few important points in mind. Here, we've listed out some of the most important things to be kept in mind.

✓ Never use your hands for leverage. This can result in serious back and neck problems.

✓ Use your hands only to keep the head stable and still.

✓ Keep your knees flexed. If you keep your legs totally straight, then there is an excess of pressure on the base of the spine.

✓ Stop the workout immediately if you feel discomfort in any of the muscles and spinal areas except the abdominals.

✓ Remember to inhale as you get up and exhale as you come back to the floor.

✓ Make sure you perform the workout without any jerks. Smooth movement through out the exercise is the key.

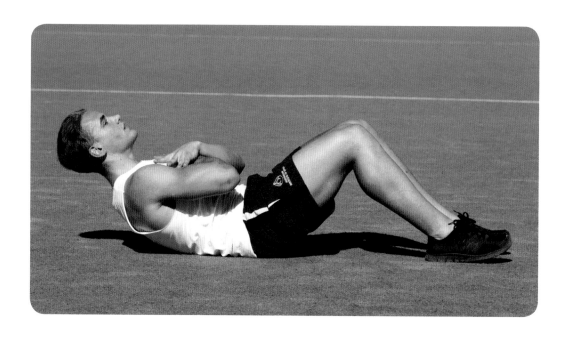

THE METHODOLOGY

The 3:21 Workout follows a very systematic and organized approach for its implementation. As we explained earlier, there are 6 modules which are to be done for 30 seconds each. This will make it a total of 180 seconds or 3 minutes for the whole workout to complete.

Here is what the schedule of the 3:21 program should look like. However, you can always make relevant and required changes to the structure and sequence of the workouts.

Each of the modules has to be done for 30 seconds each, preferably in the same sequence, at least to begin with. You can choose the body region you want to focus, though all of the workouts usually target muscles all over the body. Once you are comfortable, you can try to make minor adjustment to suit your needs.

3:21 – The Methodology

TARGET AREA
UPPER BODY STRENGTH

Shadow boxing
Push ups
Star jumps
Sit ups
Squat jumps
High knee running on the spot

TARGET AREA
LOWER BODY STRENGTH

Squat jumps
High knee running on the spot
Star jumps
Shadow boxing
Push ups
Sit ups

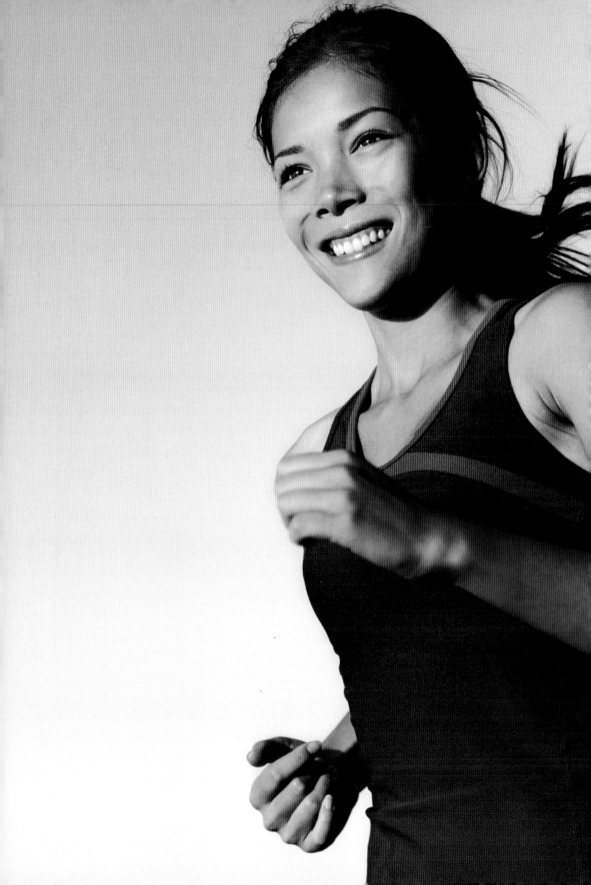

WHAT YOU MUST KNOW

The 3:21 Workout is one of the most powerful, abridged and target- based workout in the contemporary times. It follows a highly systematic and scientific approach to fitness, muscle development and other related goals.

However, such an action-packed regimen definitely comes with its own set of rules, guidelines and precautions. In this section, we've listed some of the most important guidelines to ensure that you get the best out of this amazing program.

Alongside, we've also listed a set of precautions that you must follow in order to ensure that the desired results are achieved. Read on for a detailed insight into these tips, guidelines, rules and precautions.

GETTING THE BEST OUT OF 3:21

It is an established fact that to get the best out of any venture, it is always important to devote your fullest potential to the objective. Well, fitness is no exception here. To get the best out of the 3:21 Workout, there are certain very important points or guidelines that need to be kept in mind.

Be self-motivated. No fitness program can be a success unless you don't really feel the need.

Here are some golden rules to remember if you want to get the best out of the 3:21 Workout:

1   Devote sufficient time to understanding each of the workouts in detail. As you might have seen, the 3:21 workout comprises of 6 different exercises. Each of the workouts follows a very different set of instructions and rules. This is so because each of the exercises targets a different group of muscles, Moreover, each exercise fulfils a specific fitness objective, such as core conditioning, lower body strength and conditioning and so on. Spend some time to understand what each workout means, why is it done and what is the correct way to do them. Follow the guidelines to the letter. Later, when you are very comfortable with the pattern, you can begin making some minor adjustments in accordance with your own needs.

2   Be self-motivated. No fitness program can be a success unless you don't really feel the need. Do not depend on anyone else's motivation or persistence. This fact is especially true in the case of the 3:21 Workout because the modules actually draw your maximum potential. To carry out the program effectively, you must be able to do it willingly, with all your motivation and dedication. Take your time to decide. Once you are into it, be self-motivated enough to complete it to perfection.

3   Complement your workout with other lifestyle measures. It is a proven fact that without the other supporting lifestyle changes, even such powerful programs like the 3:21 Workout fail to have the desired impact. Follow a healthy diet, exercise regularly, take proper sleep and follow all other dictates of a good lifestyle.

4   For best results, try to do the workout at the same time of the day, every day, at least for the first 21 days. This helps your body to get into the mode of exercise and sets the pattern for the daily workout.

POINTS TO REMEMBER – THE PRECAUTIONS

While the above section laid out some important rules to enable you to derive the maximum benefit of the 3:21 program, this portion talks of some important precautions that need to be observed to ensure that the set objectives are achieved. Read on for a detailed look into what all you need to keep in mind in this regard.

1 Don't let your efforts drop. The basic underlying logic of the program lies in the fact that you need to push yourself at least to the limit of 85%.Push yourself to the optimum level of 85%.

2 When you are exercising to this limit, do not continue if you feel pain or get over-exerted. Do not push yourself beyond pain in any situation. If you feel strong pain at any point, just stop and if need be, consult a health professional.

3 Do not halt the workout mid way. It has often been observed that individuals who complete the 21 at a stretch achieve much better results than those who do the 21-day schedule in parts. You will not have similar results if there is any break in the momentum.

4 Do not experiment with your shoes and the surface you exercise on. Athletes often make the mistake of using concrete or firm surfaces or wearing the wrong shoes. All of the modules in the 3:21 Workout are very high intensity and have a major impact on the knees and leg muscles. Wearing wrong shoes could damage your knees or other muscle groups in a major way.

5 Do not exercise if you've any serious health issues. For instance, most of the workouts of the 3:21 Workout can quicken the heart rate and also burn much more calories than the conventional, steady-state exercises. In such a condition, excess of exertion can actually create health issues for the individual.

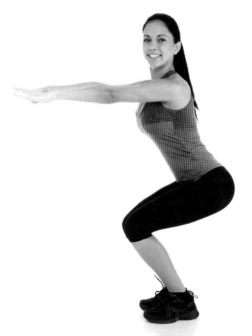

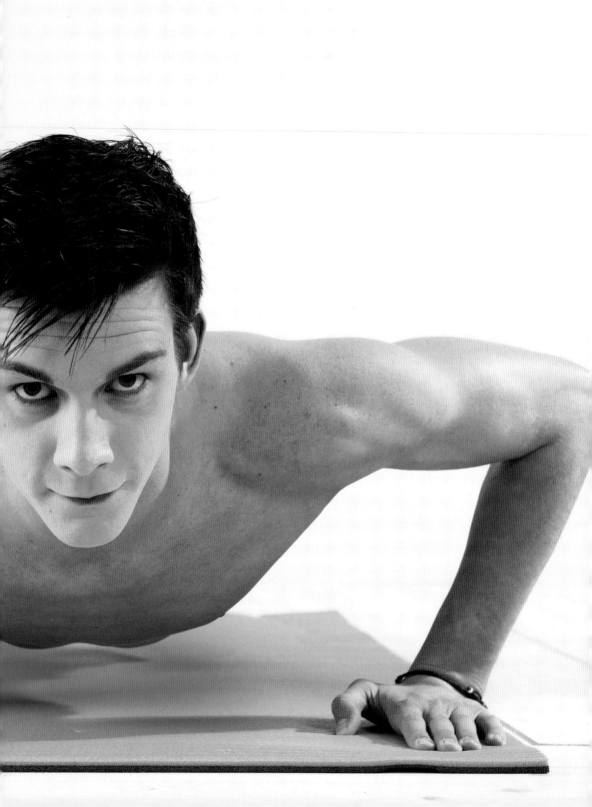

THE FUTURE AHEAD

As you progress ahead on the road to fitness, you are likely to make all-new discoveries about your own self. Modules like the squat jumps, pushups, sit-ups and shadow boxing are likely to bring out the best in you. However, you will also need to push yourself to your outer limits. This will be especially true if you have not been exercising very regularly in the past. Your muscle groups would have gone into inertia due to prolonged periods of inactivity. Just make sure you start with the 3:21 regimen in the right manner and keep up the momentum later.

Another aspect you always need to bear in mind is your lifestyle. No amount of exercise will help you unless your lifestyle complements your efforts. Make sure that you eat well and according to your own body type. You also need to give your mind and body adequate rest for a regimen such as the 3:21 to help you. In some cases, people also need psychological health services to keep themselves anxiety and stress free in today's competitive world. Just make sure all of these aspects are duly taken care of.

Only in such a case will you be able to attain the desired levels of fitness, along with physical and psychological well-being.

THE LAST WORD

Times have changed and so have we! The human body, though it remains as pristine in its structure, as it was at evolution, has also undergone a metamorphosis. Our biological systems now react to the environment in a different manner from it used to be a couple of decades back. After all, how else would anyone explain the most prominent revolutions in our societies where....

✓ The biological child-bearing age is slowly but steadily rising, giving women the much-needed space and time to devote themselves to their professional interest

✓ The average life span of an average healthy adult is increasing day by day, owing to the vast slurry of medical facilities

✓ Ironically, where the age of a cardiac arrest is rapidly falling from post 60s to post 40s.....

Well, the above are actually just a few instances give here in an attempt to show just how times are changing. With it our body's needs are also changing. While a daily round of brisk walk or a jog around the neighborhood park would suffice earlier, the intensity of exercise now has morphed beyond imagination, at least for the average healthy, middle aged adult.

More, the world of competitive sports has also undergone a sea change. With mounting pressure and heightened career goals, sportspersons hanker after expert services which can give them the much needed respite from pain and discomfort in no time.

Minimum time, maximum results, that's the dictum of the day!

The 3:21 Workout is just a step that direction. To give you, the health conscious modern day individual, just the right, power-packed fitness solution promising to address your woes and take you on a path to a newer you.....

To good health, sound fitness and a vibrant life ahead...

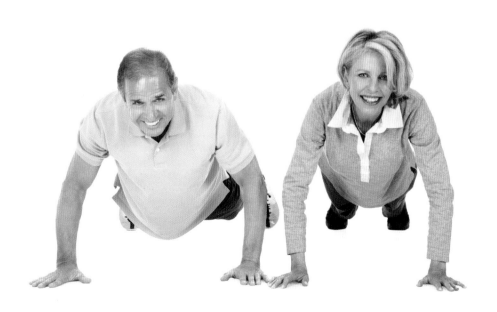

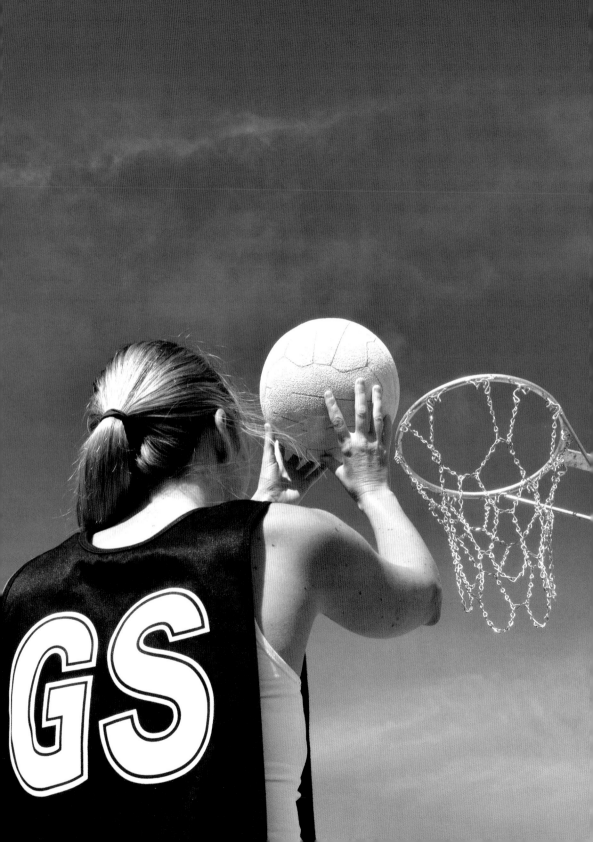

CASE STUDIES 3:21 ROUTINE

JESSICA, 24 YEAR OLD FEMALE NETBALLER

Jessica wanted a program that allowed her to maintain her gains in the gym. She played netball and wanted a workout that increased her upper and lower body strength as well as core control. She started doing the 3:21 Routine as part of her pre-season training. Six weeks into preseason she had already increased her vertical leap, court speed and agility.

> She played netball and wanted a workout that increased her upper and lower body strength as well as core control.

CHRISTINA, 48 YEAR OLD OFFICE WORKER

20 years of office work and being a single mother meant that Christina was not able to look after herself. She was 20 kgs overweight and wanted to exercise and be healthy again. She was self conscious and was reluctant to join a gym because of shyness. She started doing the 3:21 Routine from the comfort of her home. She did it for 42 days straight. Exercising everyday at such a high intensity conditioned her body and mindset. Her confidence slowly picked up – she started doing 1 class per day at the gym and then six weeks later was able to do three classes per day. After sixteen weeks she was able to lose the weight she wanted, feel great, look great and be content.

NIKKI, 14 YEAR OLD

Nikki was at an age where she was growing up and becoming self-conscious about being taller than most in her class. She experienced knee pain, shoulder pain and headaches. This was due to posture related biomechanical issues.

After her sports therapists treated the underlying biomechanical dysfunction (which took four weeks), she started the 3:21 Routine to maintain her gains. The primary plan was to improve her posture and keep her body strong and in control. The 3:21 Routine ran in conjunction with swimming every Saturday. She also loved hockey, which kept her cardiovascular system ticking along. She did modified push ups (on her knees), she loved the shadow boxing, and excelled at the squat jumps. Three months after visiting us she had better posture, no shoulder pain, minimal knee pain and she only got headaches during busy exam periods. She will continue these gains with ongoing physiotherapy and progressive exercises.

JEFF 67 YEAR OLD SOCIAL ATHLETE

A recent retiree who loves sport, Jeff continues to play tennis and swim every weekend. His wife complains that he is too fast for her when going for their afternoon walks, as he walks at 'a hundred miles an hour'. Jeff wanted to continue to build strength and improve his agility in tennis. He started the 3:21 Routine and within fourteen days he was seeing results when he played tennis. His fitness increased, he won more tennis games with ease, and found he could swim longer and faster. He was so happy that he showed his wife what he was doing and got her started with the 3:21 Routine. Although they both do the Routine together she still complains that he walks way too fast!

He started the 3:21 Routine and within fourteen days he was seeing results when he played tennis.

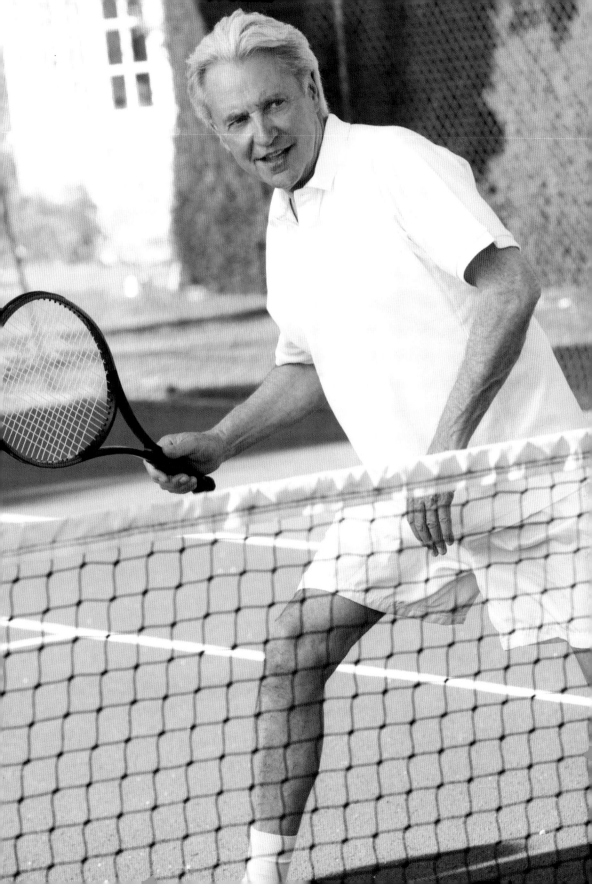

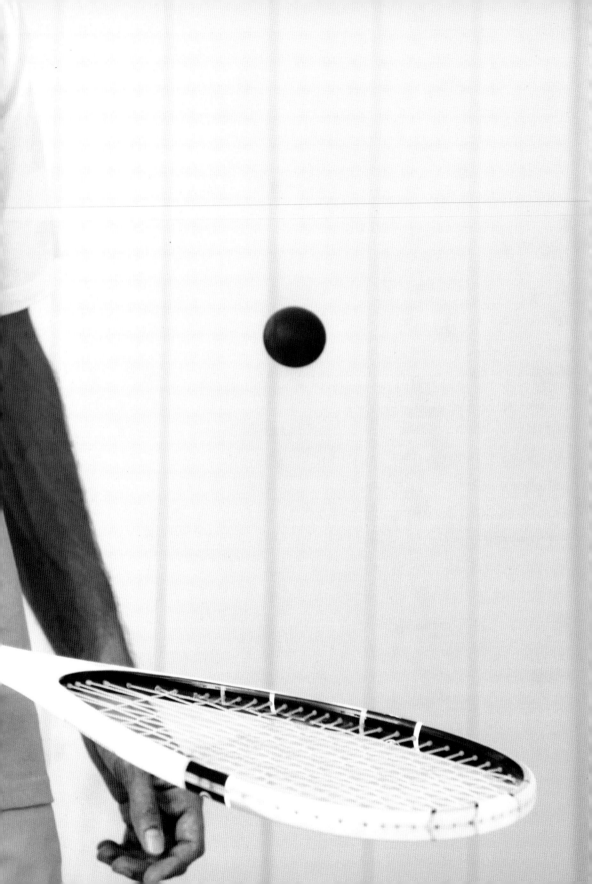

HENRY, 44 YEAR OLD EXECUTIVE

Henry travelled five days of the week. His short haul flights ranged from one to four hours. Quite an active person when at home, he missed his gym sessions and regular squash games with his friends. He started doing the 3:21 Routine to stay active when he was away. It was easy to implement in his hotel room. He started getting results in a little as fourteen days. Usually he would feel lethargic and tired with the first games of squash, and now he was able to perform at his best from the outset, last longer during rallies and win more games. Everyday niggles such as knee pain diminished to manageable levels after continuing with the 3:21 Routine every day that he was away.

Everyday niggles such as knee pain diminished to manageable levels after continuing with the 3:21 Routine every day that he was away.

JENNA, 26 YEAR OLD MOTHER

Jenna wanted to get back into exercise now that her baby was six months old. Jenna wanted to get her figure back but complications after her caesarian section meant that she couldn't exercise for twelve weeks after the birth of her baby. A sleepless child and trying to get into an exercise routine seemed impossible for Jenna. Frustrated and sad, she needed a program that was going to give her results, was safe and quick to implement, didn't require her to go to the gym and wouldn't effect her child's daily routine. Jenna started doing the 3:21 routine with the guidance of our physiotherapy team at 65% intensity. As her confidence grew, we maintained safe standards of exercise as she continued to increase her strength and core control. She used the 3:21 Routine as a stepping stone for more exercise routines including swimming and group exercise classes. For her baby's one year birthday Jenna reported that she was feeling and looking better than when she fell pregnant.

ROBERT, 33 YEAR OLD ENTREPRENEUR

Robert was an active entrepreneur, but exercise would always come second. His business needs seemed to always come first. Having a young family to support also meant that weekly football games and gym sessions would be cancelled regularly. His lack of exercise frustrated him and made Robert a grumpy man. He started the 3:21 Routine and after 21 days his body felt lighter. He felt more freedom in his movements, joints and muscles. His concentration improved and his wife said that he was less grumpy. He was able to do the 3:21 routine in his office, at home and when travelling. A happier Robert meant that he was a more effective and efficient leader for his organisation.

ELLIE, 28 YEAR OLD ELITE TRACK AND FIELD ATHLETE

Ellie travelled extensively throughout Europe and North America for her athletics needs. Whenever she travels she would end up in hotels that didn't have gyms or pools for her conditioning and recovery work. The 3:21 Routine allowed her to keep her conditioning standards up until she could get to the gyms and pools that she wanted. On some days she would do the 3:21 Routine twice because travel was that hectic.

The 3:21 Routine allowed her to keep her conditioning standards up until she could get to the gyms and pools that she wanted.

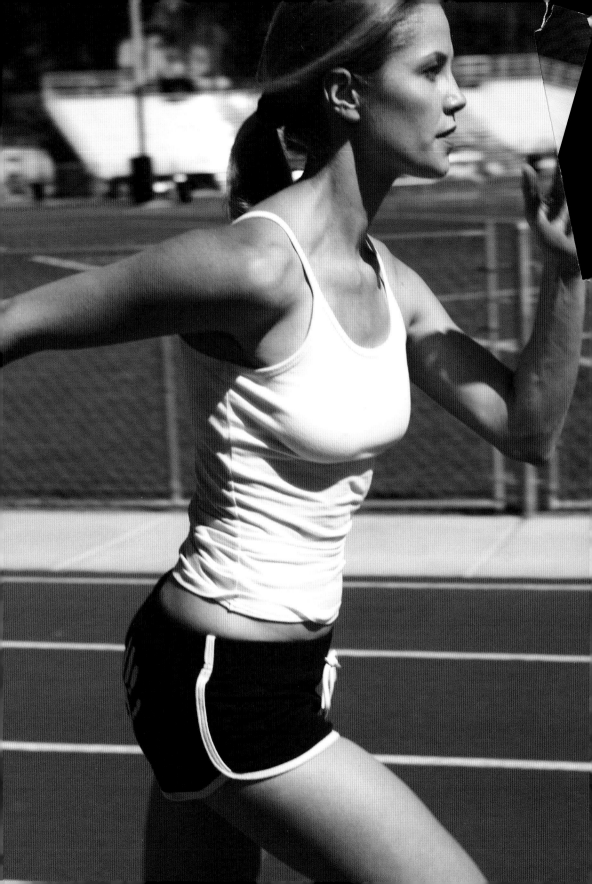

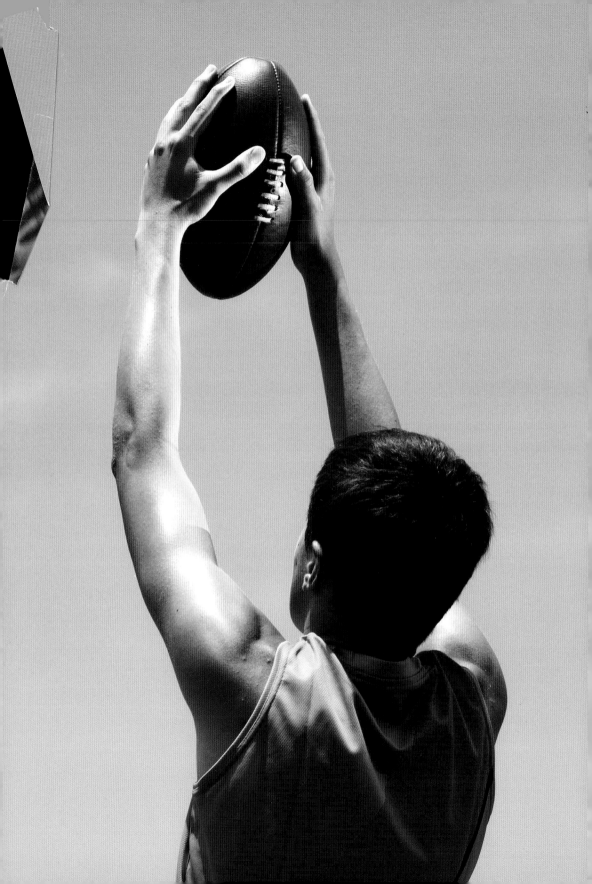

CRAIG, 16 YEAR OLD FOOTBALLER

A very active young man, Craig was accepted into the state football league. His mother came with him during his consultation and said that he had 'energy to burn' and couldn't sit still. He would train 3 times per week, attend team camps and embrace his new found level in his sport. He did the 3:21 Routine over 21 days. In 21 days his upper body strength improved and was more agile with his running drills. After 42 days his fitness levels were higher, he was training harder and he was classified to be in the top 10% in the team for vertical leap, sit and reach tests, flexibility, fitness and functional strength. From a sports therapist's perspective he had to be monitored closely for the first 21 days and thereafter every five days so he didn't push himself above levels that he couldn't tolerate. Sometimes young athletes can be head strong and they feel that they can conquer the world. They have to be held back for their own good and for them to achieve their best results.

AMY, 25 YEAR OLD

Amy was planning a family. However doctors advised her that she needed to lose 10kg otherwise she would be in a high risk category for gestational diabetes. On a mission to lose weight she wanted something she could do everyday between gym sessions, pump and pilates classes. She added the 3:21 Routine as a top-up after her gym sessions. With regular exercise, a monitored diet and a structured exercise program, she lost the required 10kgs in twelve weeks. Amy's doctors were happy that she was less likely to get gestational diabetes, and so was she.

He did the 3:21 Routine over 21 days. In 21 days his upper body strength improved and was more agile with his running drills.

INDEX

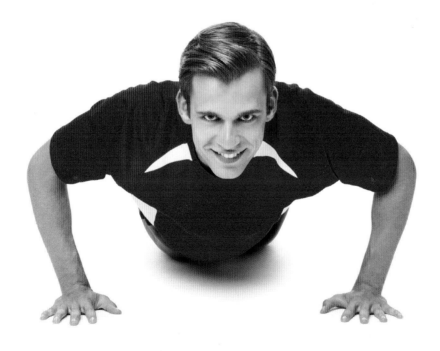